Penny, Annlee + Mercy,
You each remain in my heart
and prayers. May the Beloved
bless your family with all the love
and hope you will ever need
for the journey.
Love
Joshua

Order this book online at www.trafford.com
or email orders@trafford.com

Most Trafford titles are also available at major online book retailers.

Note for Librarians: A cataloguing record for this book is available from Library
and Archives Canada at www.collectionscanada.ca/amicus/index-e.html

Printed in Victoria, BC, Canada.

ISBN: 978-1-4269-0190-4

*Our mission is to efficiently provide the world's finest, most comprehensive book publishing
service, enabling every author to experience success. To find out how to publish your book, your
way, and have it available worldwide, visit us online at www.trafford.com*

Trafford rev. 10/9/2009

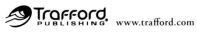 www.trafford.com

North America & international
toll-free: 1 888 232 4444 (USA & Canada)
phone: 250 383 6864 ♦ fax: 812 355 4082

Uncommon Hope

A DVD Enhanced Curriculum Reflecting the Heart of the Church for People Affected by HIV/AIDS

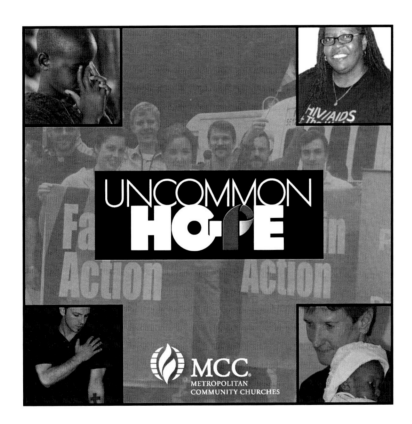

Joshua L. Love
and the Metropolitan Community Churches Global HIV/AIDS Ministry

www.uncommonhope.org

Visit the website for details about receiving the DVD component of this curriculum or information about large-print reproductions.

Lovingly dedicated to

the children of

Mother of Peace Orphanage.

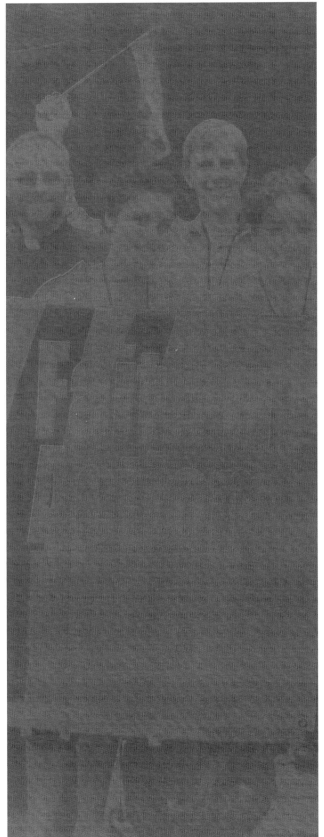

TABLE OF CONTENTS

Inaugural International March Against Homophobia,
Stigmatization & Discrimination, Mexico City, August 2, 2008

FOREWORD BY REV. DR. DONALD E. MESSER

In 1981, I became President of the Iliff School of Theology in Denver. That same year, as I grew into my new leadership role, I sought out local pastors to learn about their churches' missions and ministries and to determine how the seminary could be supportive. One of the pastors I met was Rev. Charles Arehart of the local Metropolitan Community Church (MCC) of the Rockies in Denver. We became friends and during the beginning years of the AIDS pandemic I saw MCC take faithful and compassionate action serving people who were living with AIDS.

I was asked to give a sermon at a church conference about HIV and AIDS in those early days of the AIDS pandemic. In preparation for that sermon, I asked permission to visit four or five members of MCC who were hospitalized. I shall never forget those courageous men. I told them I needed their help in writing my sermon, and they shared their stories of struggling with what then was certain death. Over and over, each individual told me, "Never give up hope." My heart was deeply moved and I have been trying to tell their stories and articulate their theologies of life and hope ever since.

MCC was addressing the HIV and AIDS crisis prior to most other Christian denominations. While others were silent or condemning, MCC was on the forefront of offering Christ's inclusive love and compassion. Today many think a faith-based response is new, but in reality Lesbian, Gay, Bisexual, and Transgender (LGBT) Christians were Christ's healers long before most Christians chose to get involved.

Those of us in other denominations (I am United Methodist) need to listen and learn from MCC, as well as express our gratitude for their selfless ministry over the years. In my travels around the world, I often remind church audiences that are often quite homophobic that we must thank God for the LGBT people who fought over the decades for antiretroviral medicine and prevention

Over and over, each individual told me, "Never give up hope." My heart was deeply moved and I have been trying to tell their stories and articulate their theologies of life and hope ever since.

education. Because of their courageous challenge to "Act Up" and reach out, millions of people have been blessed with a chance to live in the world today.

In Joshua L. Love, MCC has an articulate and winsome Christian spokesperson and leader. I am delighted to partner with Joshua and the MCC in the battle against HIV and AIDS in the world. This superb curriculum, *Uncommon Hope*, will bless both your life and your faith-based organization.

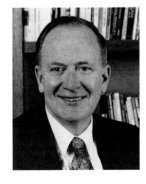

Rev. Dr. Donald E. Messer

Executive Director of the Church and Global AIDS and Author of

Breaking the Conspiracy of Silence; Christian Churches and the Global AIDS Crisis

www.churchandglobalaids.org

AUTHOR'S NOTE

The journey of HIV and AIDS transforms the world as completely as it transforms the individual. Each passing year weights our experience with an additional layer of new infections and lost lives, and like the rings of a tree, those strata bear witness to a story bigger than any single life. The sheer magnitude of the pandemic can easily overwhelm our abilities to cope, and as human capacity is exhausted, responding to HIV and AIDS becomes a walk of the spirit — a call to prayer, healing, and justice.

In the face of impossible odds, many have dared to act in order to bring the hope for an end to AIDS into the world. Even as we held our brothers and sisters in the last days of their lives and felt the potent loss of generations, our vision remained firmly set on a better day...a day when no more lives would be permanently changed by or lost to HIV and AIDS.

We believed that our seasons of lost lives and our moments of improbable physical survival held the germ of many powerful lessons. Through education, support and vision, we strove to encourage following generations to resist infection. We tried, even in our own illness, to make a difference.

Our deeply held beliefs informed our spiritual journeys and gave us tools and wisdom to share with the world. People living with and affected by HIV and AIDS searched for the deeper truths and found them — we have made a difference by stepping into the very heart of the fire to declare that God is present still among us. Now, as spiritual leaders and teachers, people living with and affected by HIV and AIDS, have a unique opportunity to heal the world as we bear witness to our own spiritual healing.

HIV and AIDS have transformed many of us in profound and powerful ways. Those whose bodies harbor the virus (a great number of us) and those who are deeply affected (almost all of us) have been challenged to grow. AIDS IS NOT OVER in the world and we have the opportunity to share what we have learned and experienced with the people who have come more recently to this path.

The impact of HIV and AIDS continues to fall most heavily on the people living at the margins of society. Viruses do not discriminate on the basis of race, ethnicity, class or sexual identity — but human beings do. Educational and medical support systems are still a privilege rather than a right for millions of people living with HIV and AIDS around the world. Communities whose members have long struggled to find equality in the world are now further burdened with rising rates of new infections, and that challenge is being met with inadequate support and social change.

What is our responsibility to the hidden and invisible people in our communities and families, to the oppressed and the powerless around us and to ourselves to the extent that we have experienced marginalization? What is our responsibility — yours and mine — to the people in our midst and around the world who are most impacted by HIV and AIDS?

Rabbi Jonathan Sacks in his 2005 book *To Heal a Fractured World: The Ethics of Responsibility*, offers the following challenge from the Jewish perspective: "We are here to make a difference, to mend the fractures of the world, a day at a time, an act at a time, for as long as it takes to make it a place of justice and compassion where the lonely are not alone, the poor not without help; where the cry of the vulnerable is heeded and those who are wronged are heard."

AIDS is an opportunity for people of faith, integrity, and compassion to say once and for all... RACISM, AGEISM, HOMOPHOBIA, HETEROSEXISM, CLASSISM, SEXISM, and all the other forms of oppression by which we subdivide our world are not acceptable anymore. The time has come for us to put an end to these evils by acting from the strength of our faith.

Local churches and faith-based organizations are often the support system of last resort for vulnerable people. A well-informed faith leader can make vital referrals and offer ongoing support to people who might otherwise "fall through the cracks" of available services. On the other hand, leaders who are not equipped with proper knowledge and understanding may, intentionally or unintentionally, broker stigmatization or evangelizing in exchange for vital services.

Because no single approach can effectively address all the root causes of vulnerability while simultaneously supporting long-term behavioral and societal changes, collaborative efforts encompassing both support and education and involving the people of both secular and non-secular organizations are required. Churches and faith-based groups comprise the world's largest volunteer base, and that base must be mobilized in order to achieve such collaboration. *Uncommon Hope* is a tool for mobilizing people of faith and promoting effective efforts to touch the lives of millions.

I hope that the material in *Uncommon Hope* will touch your life and support you in your journey of transformation. May justice, hope and healing bless your life.

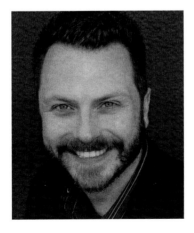

Joshua L. Love
Director of Metropolitan Community Churches
Global HIV/AIDS Ministry

www.uncommonhope.org

INTRODUCTION

***Millions of lives and millions of deaths around the world bear direct witness to
the fact that AIDS IS NOT OVER.*** The suffering and marginalization of people living with and
affected by HIV and AIDS has continued for three decades without ceasing.

+ What does this mean for people of faith and communities of faith?

+ What does it mean when people called to mercy, compassion and justice stand
  inactive, or worse, contribute through judgment and exclusion to the stigmatization
  of and discrimination against people living with HIV and AIDS?

+ How has this separation from people who are suffering worked to disconnect
  faithful people from the Divine?

+ For the faithful few, who for thirty years have been serving people living with and
  affected by HIV and AIDS, what does it mean to live in a faith-based community that
  is now waking up to a long-neglected ministry?

Uncommon Hope offers a dynamic curriculum for small groups to facilitate spiritual exploration
and formation as well as general awareness and education. Whether you are a seasoned activist
or just discerning your need to step forward, ***Uncommon Hope*** will provide tools and action steps
to support your faithful response. We all have to work together to bring about an end to AIDS.

At Metropolitan Community Churches we believe God is calling people of faith to end the silence
and inaction which have hurt millions of people around the world. We believe that silence
and inaction, particularly in the face of the human suffering and death wrought by HIV and AIDS,
are contrary to the expressed core teachings of all major faith traditions. Metropolitan
Community Churches have stood at the forefront of the battle since the first announcements linking
HIV and AIDS with the lives of gay men. We believe that God has uniquely called people of
faith to restore the heart of the church through ministry with those individuals most excluded by
the church.

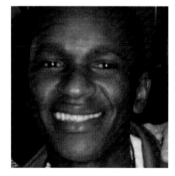 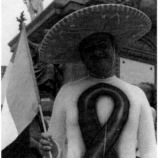 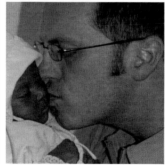 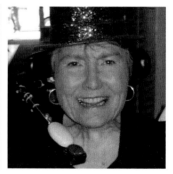

If you hunger to minister at the true intersection of justice, mercy, compassion and hope, then read these pages. The God of your understanding may be inspiring and empowering you with the message once delivered by St. Teresa of Avila:

God has no body now on earth but yours.
Yours are the only hands with which God can do work;
Yours are the only feet with which God can go about the world;
Yours are the only eyes through which God's compassion can shine forth upon a troubled world.

St. Teresa, 1515-1582

+ Will you serve as the healing hands of a loving God in the lives of people infected and affected by HIV and AIDS?

+ Will you join the passionate workers for justice who have, in the words of Rev. Troy Perry, Founder & 1st Moderator of Metropolitan Community Churches, "put feet to our prayers," in the collective effort to end the AIDS pandemic?

+ Will you make a difference because your compassion, your faith, and your hunger for justice compel you to do so?

Uncommon Hope helps communities to understand the history and complexity of HIV and AIDS while supporting people of faith to develop their own best responses and practices, to strategize community actions and to take concrete next steps by:

+ Increasing awareness and understanding of the realities of HIV and AIDS within the participants' immediate constituency, in the local community, and around the world;

+ Encouraging each participant to respond to the pandemic in at least one way;

+ Empowering people living with and affected by HIV and AIDS not only to live positively, but also to develop as advocates of spiritual growth and change within faith-based organizations;

+ Inspiring spiritual growth through remembering our history with HIV and AIDS and projecting our future toward the time when a cure will be found and AIDS WILL BE OVER;

+ Facilitating dialogue between people of many unique perspectives and experiences because in the world today we are all affected by HIV and AIDS;

+ Creating social support networks that are organic to the communities where they are most sustainable;

+ Addressing and ending the "conspiracy of silence" born of stigma, shame, and discrimination which prevents open dialogue.

OVERVIEW OF THE CURRICULUM

Whether your church or faith-based organization is just beginning to engage in HIV and AIDS ministry or has a long history in the work, this ministry program offers tools and experiences to help you develop a vital, spiritual response that is both authentic to your community and respectful of the rich diversity of human lives impacted by the HIV and AIDS pandemic.

Uncommon Hope is open and inclusive of all people living with HIV and AIDS, whether they are infected in the body or affected as concerned and caring community members. The program is a progressive, multi-unit curriculum packaged in six chapters that can be addressed by the group according to the needs of the participants. Although the curriculum is organized sequentially, each unit can stand alone and the completion of earlier units is not a prerequisite to deriving benefit from later ones. Each unit is a combination of educational tools, engaged learning, public action, and social support. The participants will be afforded the opportunity to acquire new skills and insight at each stage of the process: *Awareness, Truths, Radical Change, and Inspiration.*

Awareness

The experience of HIV and AIDS is a journey of the body, mind and spirit that transforms the lives and realities of individuals, families, communities, economies and our world. It challenges the limits of human endurance and resourcefulness. From its initial appearance as a poorly understood killer of the marginalized, to its current manifestation as a catalyst for destructive change in millions of lives around the globe, AIDS, along with HIV, has required a deep and wrenching engagement with our physical, emotional and spiritual resources.

Responding to HIV and AIDS challenges us to confront Poverty, Racism, Classism, Sexism, Heterosexism and Ageism, to name but a few of the factors which contribute to marginalization. Where these factors have been allowed to thrive, rates of HIV infection increase.

Truths

HIV and AIDS ARE NOT OVER. The global impact of HIV and AIDS rivals and exceeds that of wars and natural disasters: more than 25 million deaths; more than 33 million people infected with the virus and still living.

Three decades into our journey with HIV and AIDS, *THERE IS NO CURE.*

Medical treatment improves the lives of those with access to care, but the majority of people living with the disease in the world today do not have that access. For many, the support of a spiritual community may be the most important, if not the only, external resource they have.

Radical Changes

HIV and AIDS alter people's relationships with their bodies, their families and their faith communities — even their core beliefs may be affected. Radical acts of healing and restoration are necessary. HIV and AIDS are life-defining experiences and no single set of strategies, supports, actions and spiritual formation is appropriate or even workable for each affected individual. Furthermore, each individual's unique and dynamic journey will engender different needs and require different responses at different stages of the person's walk with HIV and AIDS.

Inspiration

Traveling the path of HIV and AIDS requires a walk of the spirit, an exploration of faith, and a confrontation of our most palpable humanity. While it is true that much has been lost to HIV and AIDS, it is also the case that much has been gained as a consequence of our powerful adaptive responses over the span of the journey. We grow closer to one another and to God as a result of compassionate and justice-based HIV and AIDS ministry and activism.

HIV and AIDS serve as a refiner's fire for many of us — baser elements that might divide us are burned away leaving hope and a shared strength that bind us together.

As people of faith we stand poised to take our next steps. It is our ***Uncommon Hope*** which *increases* our strength and keeps HIV and AIDS from overwhelming us as the journey continues. Together we walk towards the day when AIDS WILL BE OVER.

Remembering the many of our number who lost their lives to HIV and AIDS serves a vital role in the healing of our communities. Our tears cleanse weary hearts, release toxic anger, and remind us of our precious humanity. Speaking the names aloud in private meditation, at World AIDS Day commemorations or in our communities, frees us to grieve in order to make possible the work we are called to do to bring an end to HIV and AIDS. The approximately 1000 names you see listed in this publication are the first wave of submissions to the MCC AIDS Memorial. They represent only a fraction of the members, friends and family of MCC whose deaths have been AIDS-related. We remember these men, women, and children. We remember the many whose names are lost to us. And we honor also the numberless multitude who have no one left to remember them.

Greg Abbe	Fred B.	Thomas Benson	Richard Brooks	Marcos Calixto	Dewey Childs
Wat Abbot	Paul Backus	Wesley Benton	Aurthur Brosky	Rick Callahan	Casey Chisholm
Donald Abbott	Benny Bacley	Jack Berands	Michael Brousard	W.A. Callaway	Bill Chown
Fred Abercrombie	Charlie Bacon	Rev. Ron Bergeron	Jimmie Brown	Rev. David Callentine	Ron Ciolli
Jim Adams	John Bahr	Mark Bergman	Kenny Brown	Dale Cambel	Bill Clark
Lew Adams	David Bailey	Stuart Bermudez	Erik Browning	Michael Cameron	Boe Clark
Vic Adams	Joan E. Baker	Robert Berry	Michael Brumfield	Cynthia Campbell	Christopher Clark
Tommy Adcock	Daven Balcomb	James Bertram	Dr. Larry DuRand Brunson	Dallas Canada	George Clark
Bill Addy	Brian Ball	Anore Beverly	Stacey Brunson	Mark Cardwell	David Clarkson
Joe Alcantar	Houston Ball	George Bihlmeye	Rev. Grant Brush	Craig Carlan	Scott Cleaver
Eric Alderman	Fritz Baily	Rod Bingham	Mark Bruzzese	David Carlin	Steve Clement
Charles Allen	Tom Banforth	Keith Bishop	Jimmy Bryan	Dan Carlson	Douglas Clements
Genye Allen	David Baraby	Scott Bishop	Robert Buchanan	Bill Carr	Don Clenard
Gregory Allen	John Barber	Rev. Carl Bivens	Evan Buck	Bob Carter	Richard Clot
Dan Alley	Peter Barchi	Vern Black	Russell Budd	Ivan Lee Carter	Steve Clover
Jeffrey Alan Alons	Bill Barr	Sunshine Blaker	Steve Budd	Nicholas Carter	Angela Clumack
Fred Alvidrez	George Barr	Rev. Ken Bland	Doug Bull	T. Randy Carter	Mike Clumack
Michael Amaro	Ken Barr	Bill Bloomer	Roger Bullis	Craig Carver	Charles Cobb
Reynaldo Ameixeiro	Ruben Barrera	Paulo César Bonfim	Bill Bunce	Miguel Casanova	Frank Cochierra
Bert Amlung	Robert Barrows	Jim Bontrager	Bud Bunce	David A. Castagna	Jim Cockerham
Terry Amos	Steven Barsky	Robert Booth	Bruce Bunger	Ken Caton	Fernando Codina
David Anderson	Barry Bass	Melvin Boozer	Don Burdick	Jack Cauffman	Steve Cohen
Donald Anderson	Tony Basse	Derick J. Boss	Bob Burns	Bob Causon	Brent Cole
Herky Anderson	Leslie Jacob Bates	Charles Botts	David Burns	Phillip Jordan Cauthen	Richard Cole
Kevin Anderson	Michael Bauerle	Larry Boyd	Lee Bush	Jerry Chaffee	Dennis Colella
Marvin Anderson	Phillip Bayne	Bill Boyles	Art Byers	Mark Chalmers	Michael Collins
Rev. Brad Anderson	Frank Beard	Darrell Bradley	Wayne Byrd	Danny Chandler	Ken Colter
Baby Anthony	John Becker	Ron Braithwaite	Chris Byren	Theodore (Ted) A. Chandler	Sean Colvin
Keith Apple	Charles Beebe	Paul Breton	Neil Byrne	Elmer Lee Chaplin	Frederick Combs
Felix Armas	Eddie Beeker	Bob Brewer	Randy C.	Dennis Chappelle	Brian Conaway
Mark Armbruster	Lloyd Behler	Tom Briggs	R. Cadero	Len Cheaky	Douglas J. Connolly
Jesse Arranda	Ladon Bell	Gary A. Brigham	Ralph Cahall	Tim Cherry	David Cooley
Bryan Ashby	Fred Bengay	Andre David Brooks	Charlie Cahoon	Joseph Chiaffa	Shelby Cooper
Ray Austin	Dan Bennett	Michael Brooks	John Calhoun	Chet Childers	Danny Cornelius

CHRONOLOGY

Remembering the events in the world and
in the life of Metropolitan Community Churches
as we face HIV/AIDS

+ 1959

An African man dies.
Nearly 40 years later, researchers will find HIV-1 in samples of his blood
and declare his the first known AIDS death.

+ 1969

A teenaged prostitute
with Kaposi's sarcoma dies in the USA.
In approximately 30 years researcher will trace the first U.S. AIDS case to this individual.

+ 1981

The US Centers for Disease Control (CDC)
reports 5 independent cases of pneumocystis pneumonia in gay men who are otherwise healthy.

The New York Times
prints the first mass media story on what will later be known as AIDS.

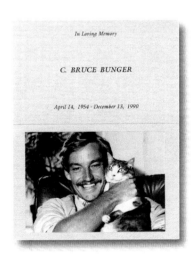

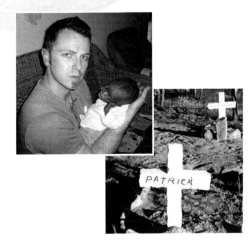

+ 1982

The CDC begins
to refer to the new disease by the more accurate
name "acquired immune deficiency syndrome."

AIDS is linked to blood
and 4 risk groups are identified: gay and
bisexual men, injection drug users, hemophiliacs,
and Haitian natives.

Six men, all private citizens,
form Gay Men's Health Crisis in New York.

The first AIDS cases
are reported in Africa.

The first case of AIDS
resulting from a blood transfusion is documented.

Sweet Spirit MCC, under the leadership of
Rev. Jodi Mekkers, is instrumental in the formation
of an AIDS rap group. The group eventually
becomes Mid-Oregon AIDS Support Services, Inc.

+ 1983

Members of high risk groups
are urged not to donate blood.

Luc Montagnier at the Pasteur Institute
in France isolates the retrovirus
(eventually called HIV) that causes AIDS.

The Denver Principles,
a manifesto of self empowerment,
is promulgated by a group of people living with AIDS.
The same group then founds the
National Association of People With AIDS (NAPWA).

Rev. Ken Martin's article "AIDS: A Pastoral, Ethical
Response" is published in *Journey*, a magazine
of the MCC's General Conference, edited by Dr. Paula
Schoenwether.

+ 1984

Despite community protests,
San Francisco officials close the city's
gay bathhouses and sex clubs.

Rev. Steve Pieters' writes "AIDS: A Gay Man's Health
Experience" in which he details his diagnosis and
medical care. The article, which humanizes the experience
of living with AIDS and calls on churches to step fully
into AIDS ministry, is published in *Journey*.

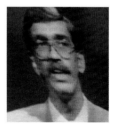

The first HIV antibody test
is approved by the US Food and Drug
Administration (FDA).

Blood banks begin to screen
donations for HIV.

The first International AIDS Conference
is held in Atlanta, Georgia (USA).

The American Foundation for AIDS Research
(AmFAR) is founded, with Elizabeth Taylor
as national chairwoman.

Public awareness of AIDS increases
with the announcements of actor Rock Hudson's
illness and subsequent death.

The first made-for-TV movie
to focus on AIDS, *An Early Frost*, airs in the US.

AIDS cases are reported
on every populated continent.

US Surgeon General Dr. C. Everett Koop,
issues a report calling for public health
measures and sex education to combat
the growing epidemic.

The first panel
of the **NAMES Project AIDS Memorial Quilt**
is created.

Supermodel Gia Carangi dies
of AIDS-related complications.

In the USA alone,
cumulative AIDS cases number 42,355 and
deaths add to 26,710.

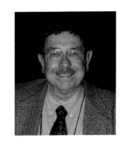

Rev. David Farrell and MCC San Diego (California,
USA) host a 50-hour AIDS Vigil of Prayer. In
addition to continuous prayer, there are musical
presentations, ecumenical worship services,
awareness and education booths staffed by various
AIDS organizations, medical and legal professionals
offering the latest pertinent information from their
fields, fund raising and volunteer registration for
AIDS-related charities, and opportunities for people
with AIDS to share their experiences.

At the request of MCC Fellowship officers,
Rev. David Farrell and MCC San Diego make the
50-hour AIDS Vigil of Prayer both Fellowship-wide
and international. MCC San Diego creates a
comprehensive "how-to" Vigil Kit and the kit is
distributed to every church in the denomination.
MCCs around the world embrace the idea and other
churches and organizations also elect to support
the effort. When final reports and results are
tabulated, it is determined that over 5,000 churches
worldwide have participated in some way in the
50-hour International Vigil.

The MCC's Third International Christian Conference
for Lesbian and Gay People of Color addresses
the topic of AIDS Ministry in Minority Communities
with a featured speaker and several specially
focused workshops.

+1987

ACT UP
The AIDS Coalition to Unleash Power holds
its first protest in New York City.

The FDA approves the use of AZT,
the first anti-HIV medication.

The U.S. bars HIV-infected immigrants
and travelers from entering the country.

The CDC broadens the definition of AIDS;
reports based on the newer definition
better reflect the scope of AIDS impact, and
affected individuals in the USA benefit
from increased access to governmental
and societal support services.

And the Band Played On,
Randy Shilts' chronicle of the AIDS epidemic,
is published.

Legislation banning the use of tax dollars
for AIDS education materials that "promote or
encourage, directly or indirectly,
homosexual activities" is passed by the
U.S. Congress.

The FDA allows condom makers
to state on their labels that latex
prophylactics could
help prevent the transmission of HIV.

The NAMES Project
is established and the AIDS Memorial Quilt
is displayed for the first time
on the National Mall in Washington, D.C.

Rev. Steve Pieters, appointed by the Board of
Elders as MCC Field Representative for
AIDS Ministry, begins traveling throughout MCC,
preaching and teaching about AIDS.

MCC introduces *ALERT*, a monthly newsletter
containing current information regarding AIDS
legislation, education, research and treatment; the
publication is targeted primarily to individuals
involved in AIDS ministry.

MCC Brooklyn, pastored by Rev. Susan Eenigenburg,
announces the launch of AIDS Ministry services,
including pastoral and spiritual care as well as a
food pantry, for people with AIDS living in Brooklyn,
New York (USA).

Rev. Elder Don Eastman represents MCC on an
AIDS National Interfaith Network (ANIN) formed in
Washington D.C.

Divine Redeemer MCC in Glendale, California (USA)
establishes a religious order, the Missionaries of
Mercy, led by the pastor, Rev. Stan Harris, to assist
AIDS patients.

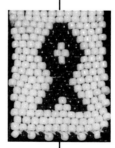

The brochure "Understanding AIDS" is mailed to each of 107 million homes in the USA.

The National Institutes of Health (USA) establishes the Office of AIDS Research and the AIDS Clinical Trials Group.

World AIDS Day is observed for the first time.

The AIDS Memorial Quilt tours 20 U.S. citites. Panels are added in each city and number more than 6000 by the end of the tour.

The first CDC guidelines for the prevention and treatment of pneumocystis pneumonia are issued.

After 2 years of protests, the manufacturer lowers the price of AZT by 20%.

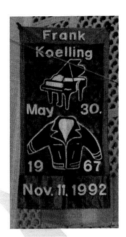

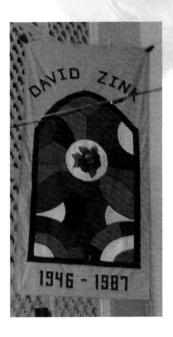

+ 1989

MCC is in the forefront of the Interfaith Movement in the USA when a number of MCC representatives participate in *AIDS – The Moral Imperative: A Call to National Leadership,* at which more than 100 religious leaders gather to discuss a unified religious community response to the challenges posed by AIDS. Participants discuss and sign on to the "Atlanta Declaration," which calls for creative action from all institutions – medical, social, economic, political, and religious – for the purpose of providing comprehensive attention to the HIV epidemic.

Richard Haller
Carol Halper
John Halpin
Neil Hamilton
Ric Hand
Rev. Brian J. Hanlon
Dean (Cory) Hansen
Deborah Hardy
Bernard Harkin
Michail Harner
Craig Harnett
Joe Harper
Michael Harrington
Rev. Jim Harris
Virgil Harris
Greg Harrison
Inock Harrison
Carl Harvey
Wendell J. Harvey
Vaughn Hayden
Mike Healy
Ed Helms
Dirk Henderson
Paul Henderson
John F. Hennessey, Jr.
Rev. Jack Herman
Sergio Hemandez
Patrick Leo Herndon
Bill Herter
Joe Hesketh
James Highiand
Rene Highway
Rev. H. Byron Hilbun
Frank Hildenbrandt
Mike Hill
Peter Hill
Rev. Bruce Hill
Rev. Randall Hill
Sam Hill
Ed Hitsman
John Hobert
Bill Hocker
John Hocking
Michael Hodges
Michael Hoffman
Michael Hogan
Rufus Hogan
Sean-Patrick Hogan
Jim Hohman
Ross Holits
Dana Holland

Rev. David Holzhauer

Tim Hoover

Harlan Hopper

Dennis Hoppes

Stephen Hostetler

Doug House

Mack Howard

Scott Howell

Keith Howey

Hal Hudson

David Huggins

David Hughes

Kevin Hull

Phil Hunt

Richard Huston

Picie Hylton

William Ingersoll

Jen Isner

Amani Jabari

Chris Jackson

John Allen Jacobs

George Jardert

Patricia Jarman

Jeff Jeffers

Jerry Ray Jernigan

Larry Jetter

Francis Joachim

Robert Johanningmeier

Jim Johner

B.J. Johnson

Casey L. Johnson

Dana Johnson

Gary Alen Gram Johnson

Jay Johnson

Jeff Johnson

Joe Johnson

Joseph Johnson

Scott Johnson

Fred Johnston

Walter Johnston

Lon Johson

David Jones

Donald Jones

Ken Jones

Len Jones

Mark S. Jones

Rev. Bob Jones

Rev. Carlos Jones

Ritchie Jones

Bill K.

Randy K.

+ 1990

18-year-old hemophiliac Ryan White,
whose case had come to symbolize the
intolerance shown to HIV-positive people,
dies 5 years after receiving
an HIV-tainted blood transfusion.

The first National Conference
on Women and AIDS is held in the U.S.

AIDS activists boycott
the Sixth International Conference on AIDS
in San Francisco
in protest of the U.S. ban on HIV-positive visitors.

Longtime Companion,
the first feature film to deal with the impact of AIDS
on friends and families, is released.

Several MCC congregations in California (USA) report AIDS ministries that have been operational for 2 to 4 years. MCC Los Angeles, MCC of the Pomona Valley, MCC Long Beach, Divine Redeemer MCC, and MCC in the Valley offer varied services—direct care, counseling, food banks, hospital/home visitation, domestic assistance, etc.—and all of the churches are actively involved in strengthening and extending their ministries.

Sixty-five persons from around the USA, Canada and the U.K. attend MCC's Second Samaritan College AIDS Conference in Houston, Texas. Conference participants are enthusiastic about the presenters and content of the conference, and many people report that the information delivered in the Medical Update has allowed them, for the first time, to understand the challenges that AIDS poses to the medical community.

MCC Kansas City (Missouri, USA) dedicates a new facility that will allow an expansion of their already multi-faceted AIDS ministry. Components of the ministry include counseling services, a visitation program and a new walk-in center for HIV-challenged individuals.

MCC Toronto (Ontario, CAN) responds to the AIDS crisis by hiring an individual to work as a full-time coordinator for its AIDSCARE program.

MCC San Francisco, in response to a need identified by people living with AIDS, announces the organization of "Reach Out Clusters" as a way to deepen support, friendship and care for and among persons living with AIDS.

In a denomination-wide survey, 45% of MCC Church Groups report numbers of AIDS-related deaths, persons living with AIDS and HIV+ individuals. Based on the data gathered, it is estimated that the denomination has experienced 4,500 deaths from HIV/AIDS, and that there are currently 2,350 congregants living with full-blown AIDS and 2,850 members who are HIV-positive.

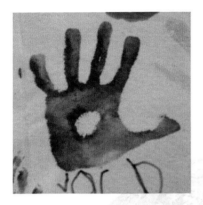

(1990 continued)

MCC Richmond (Virginia, USA) creates a new AIDS ministry, MCC CARES, which provides direct patient care, meal assistance, transportation, companionship and compassion to clients. Shortly after beginning to offer services, CARES is awarded a Certificate of Appreciation by Richmond AIDS Ministry.

Rev. Steve Pieters, Field Director of MCC AIDS Ministry, is profiled in Michael Callen's *Surviving AIDS*, the first book to address both the possibility and the reality that some people are surviving with AIDS. He is also featured in the December issue of *LIFE Magazine* which is themed "The Face of God."

✦ 1991

The Third Annual MCC HIV/AIDS Conference, focusing on HIV among people of color, is held in Orlando (Florida, USA) and is co-sponsored by MCC's AIDS Ministry and MCC's Department of People of Color. The conference offers a number of workshops, plenaries, meetings and worship services, and includes discussions confronting the issues of racism head-on.

Rev. Steve Pieters is profiled in a segment of the NBC Sunday night program "Real Life with Jane Pauley." In addition to an extensive interview with the primary subject, the segment includes film clips of Rev. Pieters engaged in various aspects of AIDS ministry with local groups at MCC Los Angeles and MCC Pueblo (Colorado, USA).

Rev. Pieters' book, *I'm Still Dancing!* in which the author is "extraordinarily honest in chronicling his own struggles with fear, anger, pain, homophobia and despair," and in which he reflects on the question, "How can I explain the miracle of my health?" is published.

MCC's General Conference XV in Phoenix, Arizona (USA) opens with a memorial service. The AIDS programming at the conference, which includes multiple workshops, a luncheon, support group meetings and a rest area for persons with AIDS, draws uniformly positive reviews.

Rev. Dr. Karen Ziegler, formerly pastor of MCC New York, founds AIDS Interfaith New York, the first stand-alone interfaith network in New York City to be directed specifically toward AIDS.

Partially in response
to the case of Kimberly Bergalis, who claimed she was infected by her dentist, the CDC recommends restrictions for some HIV-positive health care workers.

Professional basketball player Magic Johnson
announces that he is HIV-positive.

Ten years into the epidemic,
cumulative AIDS cases in the US number 257,607 and deaths total 159,818.

Grayne Kam
Richard Karikas
Gary Katz, MD
Jerry Kaufman
Tom Kay
Ed Keller
Ralph Kennedy
Michael Kenney
John Kenyon
Joe Kielwein
Joseph Killian
Rich Killingsworth
David King
James R. King
Roy King
Shawn Kinney
Lindsay Kirk
Shannon Kitzman
Gary Klink
Dan Knight
Mark Knodell
Richard Knoll
Bill Knox
Doug Koeling
Charles Kopp
Chas Korpics
Robert Kraus
Bob Krause
Darren Krause
Rodolpho Krestan
David Krumroy
Ronnie L.
Bobbie LaBelle
Dana Labnon
Karl Lack
Kevin LaClaire
Kevin Lally
Gean Lalonde
Jeff LaLonde
John Lalulya
Tom Lambert
Marty Lamica
Patrick A. Landon
Rick Lane
Gary Lanham
Stephen Lanphier
Robert Larkin
Kevin Larrabee
Father Bob Laughery
Allan Dale Law
Bill Leavens

Peter LeBhone

Dusty Leigh

Brandon Lejeune

Stephin Lemlin

Stephen M. Lenton

Deacon Chris Lentz

Michael Lentz

Randy Leonard

Manuel Lepp

Michael D. Leroux

Gary Lewis

Ken Lewis

Rev. Calvin Lindley

Tom Lindsey

Leon Linfoot

David Ray Linger

Chuck Linton

Martin Lipp

Richard D. Littlefield

Professor Jose Llompart

Warren Locke

Gabe Lopez

Larry Lord

Joe Lorh

Martin Lounsberry

Joe Loverix

Steve Loverix

Mike Lowe

Corey Lowther

Jim Lucas

Norm Luers

Bill M

Marty MacDonald

Rev. Artie MacDonald

Jim MacGregor

Skip MacGregor

Domingo Machado

Larry MacIndoo

Mario Magana

Randy Magee

George Mageean

Rev. Don Magill

Carl Magill-Knitig

Rev. Dan Mahoney

Kevin Mair

Elder Michael Mank

Mark Mann

Dave Manor

Donald Manson

Phil Manthei

Christopher Manuel

AIDS becomes the top killer
of American men ages 25-44.

*The CDC adopts a new set of
AIDS-defining conditions*
which includes symptoms specific to
injection drug
users and women.

The AIDS Memorial Quilt
now contains panels from every U.S. state
and 28 other countries.

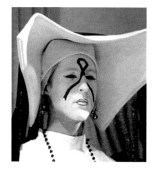

+1992

MCC's HIV/AIDS programming in Dallas, Texas (USA) encompasses multiple support groups, professional counseling services, the *Care Bears* care-giving teams, hospital visitation volunteers, and the provision of the only emergency funds available to persons with HIV/AIDS in the city. Cathedral of Hope MCC is honored by AIDS Services of Dallas for their "outstanding contributions" to the AIDS House, where fifty men, women and children with HIV/AIDS live.

After more than a year of preparation, Christos MCC in Toronto (Ontario, Canada) announces that the Lou Segal House Foundation will provide temporary accommodations for people coming to Toronto for medical treatment or to visit loved ones in hospital. It is expected that the facility will cater primarily to those affected by HIV, but no one facing a medical crisis will be turned away.

First MCC of Atlanta (Georgia, USA) receives an $18,000 grant to provide full-time pastoral counseling to those living with and affected by HIV. The new ministry will augment First MCC's ongoing outreach, which includes an HIV Food Pantry, Support Groups, weekly NAMES Project quilting bees, monthly food preparation for an interfaith daycare support facility, and two holiday gift basket programs.

Good Samaritan MCC in Whittier, California (USA) announces the creation of Proclamation Press, which will publish a quarterly theological journal. Proceeds from the sale of the journal, *Life in Christ,* will be used exclusively to provide scholarships for student clergy who are HIV+, have AIDS or suffer from other life-threatening illnesses.

The Long-Range Planning Task Force for MCC's AIDS Ministry, charged by the Board of Elders to conduct a needs assessment of the fellowship and to develop recommendations for future program objectives, sends AIDS Response Surveys to every church in the Fellowship.

(1992 continued)

Rev. Howard Williams, pastor of MCC Santo Domingo (Dominican Republic) reports that the government agency "Corta" has enlisted MCC in an educational outreach program targeted to street hustlers.

Agape MCC in Ft. Worth, Texas (USA) begins "Spiritual AIDS Ministry" as an outreach to provide care teams in conjunction with local interfaith AIDS services and to provide non-judgmental, non-denominational spiritual counseling to people living with HIV/AIDS.

✚ 1993

Rev. Christine Oscar and St. Mary's MCC in Greensboro, North Carolina (USA) are presented the Triad Health Project Founder's Award "in recognition of service to people living with HIV/AIDS and in recognition of an unparalleled role in acceptance of all people living with HIV/AIDS."

MCC San Francisco and MCC San Diego (California, USA) hire, respectively, an HIV Program Coordinator and an AIDS Ministry Coordinator.

The MCC AIDS Ministry publishes *The Spiritual Strength for Survival Support Group Manual*, a new resource book for local churches. The manual gives instructions on how to operate a spiritually-based support group for people with HIV/AIDS.

Rev. Elder Darlene Garner completes a term as chair of the Board of Directors of Northern Virginia AIDS Ministry. The service organization has a budget slightly less than one million dollars, serves a clientele that is 50% female, and provides numerous support services.

Rev. Jack Isbell is hired by the California Department of Corrections as chaplain for Unit 4, the HIV/AIDS Unit of the California Medical Facility at Vacaville, California (USA). He is the first MCC pastor to become a fulltime chaplain at a correctional facility.

Rev. Paul Whiting, pastor of MCC Manchester (Manchester, UK) is invited to stage a worship service with an emphasis on HIV/AIDS at the gay and lesbian festival in Manchester. It is the first time MCC has been invited to participate in the festival and the first time the festival has included a worship service.

U.S. President Bill Clinton
creates the White House Office of National AIDS Policy.

Four French officials are jailed
for allowing HIV-tainted blood into France's blood banks.

Angels in America,
Tony Kushner's play about the AIDS pandemic, is awarded the Pulitzer Prize.

The AIDS-themed film Philadelphia,
which focuses on an HIV-positive lawyer facing workplace discrimination, is released.

Victor Marino
Robert (Bob) Marko
Wayne Marple
Jim Marsh
Derek Scott Marshall
Don Marshall
Roxanne Marshall
Joseph Marsiglia
John W. Martin
Ralph E. Martin
Joesph (Tasha) Martin
Jerry Martinelli
Lino Martinez
John Masauch
Ralph Masek
Norm Mason
James Masso
Doug Matson
Douglas Matson
Carl Matthes
Tommy Mauer
Bob Mayberry
Richard Mayshock
Thomas Jay McAdams
Martin McBride
Jim McCann
Steve McCaughin
Dr. Gary McClelland
Dr. Gary McClendon
Ronald McCollam, Jr.
Ralph McCoy
Daniel McCree
Tony McCumber
Lester Peter McDonald
Sean McDonough
Larry McFarland
Jerry McGinnis
George McGovern
Robert McKeever
Mike McMahon
Rev. Don McRae
Patrick McSweeney
Fred McVey
Don Meadows
Luther Meadows
Rev. Patrick Mecham
Eddie Medina
Victor Manuel Medina
Harvey Mendelsohn
Juan Mendez
Larry Meredith

John Merick
Guy Merryman
William Mertes
Bill Mertz
Dick Mertz
Francisco Mesa
Peter Messina
Peter L. T. Messina
Sean Michael
Kevin Mielke
Wayne Mielke
Bill Miller
David Miller
Earl Miller
James Miller
Jim Miller
John Miller
Harlow Mills
Daniel Milman
Jeff Minea
Jim Minter
Scott Miording
Ron E. Miori
Marcos Mirabal
David Mitchell
Gary Lynn Mitchell
Jack Mitchell
Rev. Michael Moffatt
Norman Mogel
Steve Mohr
Don Money
Michael Montgomery
Jose Montoya
Bobby Moore
Clark Moore
David Moore
Larry Moore
Lester Moore
Paul Moore
Robert (Boby) Moore
Ron Moore
Jesus Morales
Sean William Moran
Ken Morgan
William Ray Morgan
Jerry Morrison
Rev. Cliff Morrison
Rob Morrison
Walter Morrissette
Scooter Motdoch
Bill Mueller

AIDS becomes the leading cause of death
among all Americans ages 25-44.

The U.S. Public Health Service
recommends the use of AZT to help
reduce the chances of mother-to-child
transmission of HIV during
pregnancy and birth.

The cast of the San Francisco
edition of the MTV
reality program *The Real World*
includes HIV-positive Pedro Zamora.

(1993 continued)

Victory Ministries, a Special Work of MCC's Southwest District, sends out street teams to educate people in the African-American and Latino communities of San Bernardino and Riverside Counties (California, USA) about HIV/AIDS.

Rev. Jose Marcos Gonzalez, pastor of the Latino ministry of MCC Los Angeles, is the only latino clergyperson to testify at hearings on HIV/AIDS organized by the Alianza Latino Caucus of the Los Angeles HIV Health Services Planning Council.

Rev. Elder Troy Perry, Founder and Moderator of MCC, is one of three keynote speakers at the AIDS National Interfaith Network plenary luncheon of the annual U.S. national Skills Building Conference. A participant commented, "I've never seen such a gathering of people of colors, religious people, and people living with HIV/AIDS."

+ 1994

Rev. Steve Pieters meets with President Clinton at a prayer breakfast two days before World AIDS Day. He urges the President to take action because "action creates hope." On World AIDS Day, President Clinton mentions Rev. Pieters in his speech, calling him one of America's longest survivors and explaining how Rev. Pieters stays alive through hope and his own faith.

Rev. Don Magill, an MCC clergyperson living with AIDS, instigates the publication of a monthly AIDS Newsletter for the Northwest District. The first issue features articles about women and AIDS, breast cancer and women's health resources.

MCC's AIDS Ministry program produces a new resource, "Choose Life: Taking Action To Be Fully Alive with HIV/AIDS," outlining twelve life-enhancing action steps for people living with and affected by HIV and AIDS.

Volunteers from the AIDSCARE program at MCC Toronto provide home hospice care for a great number of individuals, and the larger program now comprises the "We Care" phone contact program, the "Buddy Support" program, and the "Care Team" program.

(1994 continued)

The AIDS ministry at MCC of the Ozarks (Fayetteville, Arkansas, USA) involves at least half of the congregation's members in direct services, information services, advertising and education.

MCC Sydney (New South Wales, Australia) is offering practical support (food, clothing, and household items) as well as spiritual support and counseling to people affected by HIV/AIDS.

+ 1995

Rev. Joseph Gilbert, pastor of MCC For All the Saints in Los Angeles, is elected Chair of the Spiritual Advisory Committee of AIDS Project Los Angeles. Rev. Ralph Lasher of MCC of the Resurrection in Houston, Texas (USA) is named Program and Development Director of the Kolbe Project, a "ministry of unconditional love" which includes AIDS programming.

Joy MCC in Orlando, Florida (USA) operates an AIDS and Health Ministry, which offers outreach, education and support services, out of the Bailey Center (named for former client David Bailey) on the church's property.

MCC offers an HIV/AIDS track within the Health and Wholeness Programming at General Conference XVII in Atlanta, Georgia (USA). A number of AIDS Ministry workshops are held throughout the week and several researchers from the Atlanta-based CDC present addresses.

The Peer Education Program of the Metropolitan Community Churches announces a new HIV prevention program targeting young gay men, ages 18-25.

President Clinton
creates the Presidential Advisory Council on HIV/AIDS.

Saquinavir, the first protease inhibitor
prescribed to HIV patients, receives FDA approval.

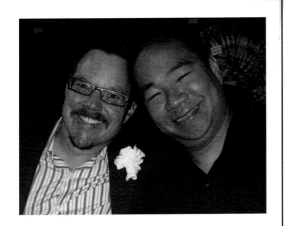

Ron Mullins
Michael Mulvaney
Charles Munoz
Daniel Munoz
James Murphy
Jimmy D. Murphy
Tobias Murphy
Rev. Frank Murr
Corky Murray
Keith Murry
Doug Muth
Francis Muto
Jackson Myers
David Napier
Troy Naranjo
Michael (Wanda Jean) Nauert
Glenn Matthew Nelson-Sterman
David Nettles
Mike Nichol
Norman E. Nichols
J. Peter Niland
Ernest Nino-Walker
John Noe
Greg Noecker
Nelson Norwood
Jeff Nuckols
Denis O'Callaghan
Tommy Ochletree
Cliff O'Connor
Richard (Rick) O'Dell
Jesse Odin
Floyd Samuel Ohler
Andy Oppy
Javier Ortega
Pete Ortega
John Ortiz
David Ostindi
Joshua O'Sullivan
Michael Otera
Martin (Steve) Owens
Bella Oyola
Jason P.
Susan P.
Victor P.
Tim Page
Michael Palmer
Greg Paludis
Robert Papp
Chip Parker
Greg Parmley

+ 1996

The Joint United Nations Programme
on HIV/AIDS is founded.

The International AIDS
Vaccine Initiative is formed.

At the 11th International Conference on AIDS,
it is reported that combination therapy,
"HIV cocktails" including protease inhibitors,
is helping extremely ill patients.

The FDA approves the first HIV viral load test.

The AIDS-themed musical Rent,
by Jonathan Larson, wins the Pulitzer Prize
and receives four Tony Awards.

TIME Magazine names AIDS
researcher David Ho, MD, Man of the Year.

After the 15th year of AIDS,
cumulative AIDS cases in the US number
611,325 and deaths total 386,046.

The AIDS Memorial Quilt
completely covers the National Mall in
Washington D.C. Because of the Quilt's size, this
is the last time it will be displayed in its entirety.

+ 1997

It is reported that AIDS-related death
fell 13 percent in the first six months of 1996,
and this first "significant" drop in deaths
since 1981 is attributed to the use of protease
inhibitors and combination therapy.

Researchers report that some HIV cells
"hide out" in specific reservoirs in the body where
they are unaffected by current drugs.

Combivir, the first multidrug pill
targeting HIV is approved.

The U.S. Congress approves a bill
to speed the FDA's drug-approval process.

MCC AIDS Ministry is awarded one of the Ryan White Youth Service Awards for the Peer Education Program.

Safe Harbour MCC of Halifax, Nova Scotia (CAN) founds *Manna for Health* in response to the growing need for food assistance among individuals with HIV/AIDS.

The Gospel Choir of MCC DC in Washington D.C. performs at a Justice Department event commemorating World AIDS Day 1996. The event marks the end of the Department's week-long AIDS awareness effort and features Jerry Foemer, a Justice Department attorney living with AIDS, Attorney General Janet Reno and others.

Positive Voices, a choir of HIV-positive men founded by Jackson Myars and associated with Cathedral of Hope MCC in Dallas, Texas (USA), receives a nomination for a GLAMA (Gay & Lesbian American Music Awards) in the choral music category.

+ 1998

African-American leaders declare an AIDS-related
state of emergency in black communities and help launch the Minority AIDS Initiative.

AIDS is no longer ranked
among the top 10 causes of death for Americans and statistical analysis shows that U.S. AIDS deaths decreased by 50% in 1997.

At the Fifth Conference
on Retroviruses and Opportunistic Infections, David Ho, MD, presents evidence that the first HIV infections probably occurred in the 1940s or early 1950s.

+ 1999

Current research indicates that HIV spread
to humans via a mutated form of a similar virus known to infect some African chimpanzees. It is thought that the simian virus may have existed for thousands of years.

The World Health Organization (WHO)
announces that AIDS has overtaken tuberculosis as the most deadly infectious disease and is now the fourth leading cause of deaths worldwide.

Strains of HIV that are highly resistant
to multiple drugs are discovered in some newly infected individuals in the U.S. and Europe.

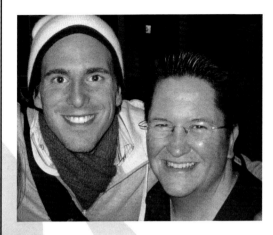

Rev. Robert Griffin, in partnership with Rev. Jim Mitulski and Rev. Elder Hong Tan, leads MCC's denominational HIV/AIDS effort. The ministry responds to the needs of individuals who, because of medical advances, now require pastoral care and leadership to regain their relationships with life rather than to cope with imminent death.

Rev. Jimmy Allen, former President of the Southern Baptist Convention, speaks to the General Conference of MCC in Los Angeles. Allen, in acknowledgement of the unprecedented nature of his appearance at the conference, tells attendees, "I felt God wanted me to be here...there's something about what God does in the human heart that reaches beyond [our] differences." He speaks about losing members of his family to AIDS and brings the crowd to its feet when he declares, "We all felt the shaft of pain to be untouchable. Nobody should be untouchable!"

+ 2000

The CDC reports that African-American and Latino men who have sex with men have higher HIV infection rates than do white men in the same transmission category.

The UN Security Council declares AIDS a global security threat.

President Clinton signs an executive order to help developing nations manufacture or import generic versions of patented antiretroviral drugs.

The Pilgrim Press publishes *Take Back the Word: a queer reading of the Bible*. MCC contributions include the chapters "Ezekiel Understands the AIDS: AIDS Understands Ezekiel, or Reading the Bible with HIV," by Rev. Elder Jim Mitulski, and "The Beloved Disciple: A Queer Bereavement Narrative in a Time of AIDS," by Rev. Robert Goss.

+ 2001

The UN General Assembly holds its first special session on AIDS.

The WTO announces an agreement to allow developing countries to make or import generic medications in the case of public health crises.

Twenty years into the AIDS pandemic, U.S. numbers for cumulative AIDS cases and deaths are 819,779 and 479,983, respectively.

+ 2002

AIDS becomes the leading cause of death across the globe for people in the age range 15 to 59.

Worldwide, about half of all HIV-positive individuals are female.

The UN-backed Global Fund to Fight AIDS, Tuberculosis, and Malaria is created.

The Metropolitan Community Foundation of San Francisco, California (USA) awards Coretta Scott King the Circles of Hope Award for her powerful advocacy and work for social justice. In accepting the award, Mrs. King praises the Metropolitan Community Foundation for having been at the forefront of advancing "...social justice for lesbian, gay, bisexual and transgendered people of all races."

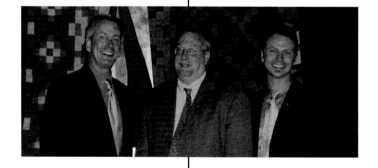

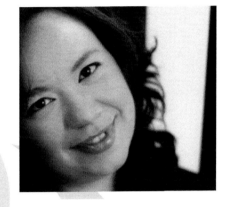

+ 2003

The FDA approves Fuzeon,
the first HIV entry inhibitor.

U.S. President George W. Bush announces
the President's Emergency Plan
for AIDS Relief to fight HIV outside the U.S.

*South Africa, which reports having
the greatest number*
of HIV-positive people in the world, announces plans
to create an antiretroviral treatment program.

+ 2004

Gilead Sciences and Bristol-Myers Squibb
announce a collaboration to combine 3 anti-HIV
drugs into a once-daily pill.

The first generic anti-HIV medication
is approved for sale in the U.S.

*Andy Bell, lead singer of the
pop group Erasure,*
announces he is HIV-positive and allows
publication of his story.

+ 2005

For the first time anti-HIV medications
are decommissioned when Roche announces
it will stop marketing Hivid and Fortovase
due to low demand.

The patent for AZT expires
and four generic versions are approved
for the U.S. market.

The WHO announces that its '3 x 5 Initiative'
—begun in 2003 to get 3 million HIV-positive
people in poor nations on
antiretroviral therapy by the end of
2005—will not reach its target.

MCC enters into a new era of Global HIV and AIDS
Ministry which includes intensive drug use and addictions
awareness, a new partnership with the Y.A. Flunder
Foundation Mother of Peace Orphanage in Zimbabwe,
and a commitment by the Board of Elders to create
of a new fulltime staff position to support the ministry.

At the General Conference in Calgary, Alberta (CAN)
Rev. Elder Jim Mitulski and Joshua Love call MCC to
demonstrate solidarity with all people living with and
affected by HIV and AIDS by wearing t-shirts printed
with the bold message HIV+. Additionally, Rev. Elder
Mitulski asks the women of MCC to stand and receive
the applause and acknowledgement of the men for
their courageous and dedicated support of the many
men who died of AIDS over the years. Love comes
out as an HIV-positive man in recovery, and commits
himself to supporting MCC in its next generation of
HIV and AIDS ministry.

Eli Staten

Jim Statt

Kenneth Steele

Don Stegeman

Darrol Stephens

Brad Stevens

Charles Stinson

Michael St'Laurant

William T. Stokes

Bill Stone

Frank Storm

David Story

Jimmy Stott

Kenneth Stouffer

Ted Straley

Mark Stratman

Jack Strejc

Stan Stroud

Alan Strunk

Greg Stuhr

Bob Stump

Kurt Stutzman

Kevin Styers

Michael Subject

Lowell Sullivan

Ron Summers

Frank Suter

Deacon Hugh Swaney

Jon Szumigala

Eddie Tamula

Jim Tanner

Bill Taylor

Cindy Taylor

Lance Taylor

Ronald Batista Tenório

John Terhune

Daniel Tessar

Garson Thomas

Steve Thomas

Dell Thompson

Wayne Tietsort

Lloyd Tittle

Bill Tobiasson

Tony Tomlin

Shelby Topp

Larry Torres

Lelano Toy

Dennis Tracy

Henry Trevathan

Chip Trotter

Roy Trussell

The U.S. Congress considers a bill shifting federal funding formulas that, if passed, will leave some of the nation's hardest-hit cities expecting ominous shortfalls in funding for public HIV resources.

In the U.S., cumulative AIDS cases now total 1,025,000 and deaths are estimated at 559,000.

(2005 continued)
Ritchie Crownfield and Alan Landis make it possible for panels of the NAMES Project Quilt to be be brought to the General Conference and lovingly displayed in worship services there.

✚ 2006

Joshua Love joins the staff of MCC as the director of the newly reformed MCC Global HIV/AIDS Ministry. He travels to local churches and conferences, visits 13 U.S. cities and journeys to Africa in order to generate awareness of the need for justice activism, comprehensive education and compassionate faith-based responses to HIV and AIDS.

At MCC's Men in Ministry conference, Rev. Steve Pieters inspires a new level of commitment to ministry in the areas of HIV and AIDS by sharing the history of the denomination's movement and work in the AIDS pandemic.

MCC Global HIV/AIDS Ministry sends a ministry team to Zimbabwe where they engage, along with representatives from the Y.A. Flunder Foundation, the United Church of Christ, Allen Temple Baptist and elsewhere, in a mission of love, respite and learning. They serve at the Mother of Peace Orphanage which houses almost 200 children, all of whom are either infected or directly affected by HIV or AIDS.

The DVD *We Who Are One Body: A Spiritual Walk with AIDS*, documents the work at Mother of Peace and becomes a rallying point from which individual MCC congregations commit themselves to AIDS ministry both locally and globally.

MCC Global HIV/AIDS Ministry begins testing a new HIV and AIDS curriculum which blends the processes of healing and memory with public calls for action and campaigns for awareness.

MCC Global HIV/AIDS Ministry begins to collect the written HIV and AIDS stories of members and allies all over the world. The stories are posted online as part of MCC's global community network, and the call for submissions from anyone living with or affected by HIV and AIDS is ongoing.

(2006 continued)

Churches raise over $40,000 (USD) in support of expanding the MCC Global HIV/AIDS Ministry; communities involved include Topeka, Tampa, Portland, Atlanta, Palm Beach, San Francisco, Las Vegas, Berkeley and others. The People of African Descent Conference and this year's Regional Conferences also contribute.

+ 2007

MCC of Greater St. Louis (Missouri, USA) receives a $50,000 grant from the Missouri Foundation for Health to establish a comprehensive program called "The Hope & Help Center" which will promote the physical, mental, and social health of lesbians, gay men, and individuals who are HIV-positive.

The MCC General Conference, held in Scottsdale, Arizona (USA), devotes an entire day of the global convocation to HIV and AIDS. Events and speakers include: an HIV and AIDS breakfast at which Rev. Elder Freda Smith urges MCC to remember its history, tell its stories and change the future; two workshop sessions at which Joshua Love leads a panel of speakers from around the world on the expansion of the MCC Global HIV/AIDS Ministry; the presentation of a special award to Rev. Robert Griffin for his passionate service to HIV and AIDS Ministry; a riveting sermon in the morning worship service in which Rev. Nokthula Dhladla illuminates AIDS from the perspective of an African woman; and an intensely moving evening worship service led by Rev. Elder Jim Mitulski in which he pairs activism and healing.

Over the course of the year, Joshua Love visits, talks, conducts workshops and/or preaches in 22 different cities in North America and Australia in connection with the work of MCC Global HIV/AIDS Ministry.

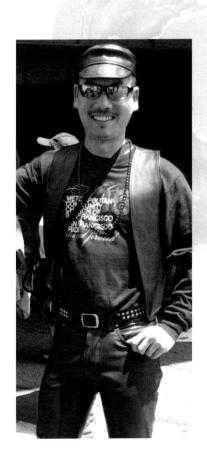

Billy Webber

Robert Weinand

Patrick Weisenburger

Rev. Joseph Welford

Rev. Howard Wells

Bob Welton

Johnny Wescott

Eric West

Len West

Don Wheatley

Gordon Wheatley

Troy Wheeler

Billy Wheless

Gregory James Wherry

Eric White

George White

Keith White

Mark White

Michael White

Rev. Woody White

Bob Wickline

Keith Wienner

David Wilcox

Dan Wilde

Wes Wilder

Joseph Wilk

William Nash Wilkinson

Alan Williams

Brian Williams

Earl Williams

James Williams

Brian Williamson

Earl Williamson

John Ray Willingham

Gary Wilson

Jim Wilson

Mark Wilson

Jimmy Wing

Michael Robert Wing

Randy Wingerter

David Wise

Keith Gordon Wismer

Robert Douglas Wolfe

Carelton Wong

Robert Wood

Bill Woods

Daniel Wornom

Gary York

Richard Young

Albert Zapata

Albert

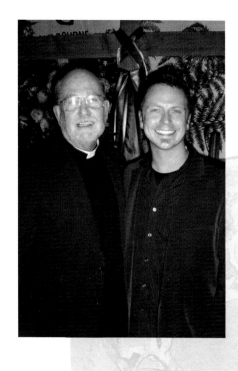

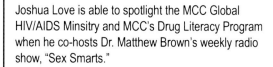

Joshua Love is able to spotlight the MCC Global HIV/AIDS Minsitry and MCC's Drug Literacy Program when he co-hosts Dr. Matthew Brown's weekly radio show, "Sex Smarts."

MCC Moderator, Rev. Elder Nancy Wilson, attends "Breakthrough: The Women, Faith, and Development Summit to End Global Poverty Conference" in Washington, D.C., at which she shares MCC's intense commitment to the issues around women with HIV/AIDS and those who are part of a sexual minority.

Joshua Love delivers the Gregory Lecture, a keynote address at Lancaster Theological Seminary. Members of the seminary and surrounding communities attend his talk as well as an afternoon workshop presentation on how churches can engage in HIV and AIDS ministry.

MCC has a distinct presence at the 2008 International AIDS Conference in Mexico City, Mexico: Joshua Love co-presents a workshop at the Ecumenical Pre-Conference with Rev. Dr. Donald Messer; Robert "Bobby" G. Pierce, a Jewish member of MCC San Francisco speaks on panel at AIDS 2008 about his experience of living with HIV and being a faith leader; Rev. Paul Mokgethi, and MCC pastor from South Africa, speaks on behalf of the International Network of Religious Leaders Living with HIV and AIDS (INERELA+); and Preben Bakbo Sloth, of Marken Liljer MCC in Copenhagen, Denmark participates in several key portions of AIDS 2008 on behalf of his secular work in HIV and AIDS, as well as his passionate commitment to MCC.

MCC undertakes to compile a list of members, friends and family whose deaths have been AIDS-related and solicits submissions from across the Denomination. The MCC AIDS Memorial is to be a dynamic, ongoing project, housed on the website *www.UncommonHope.org* and updated regularly as submissions continue.

MEMORIAL

The MCC AIDS Memorial is dedicated
to honoring our history — remembering the
individual lives of the loved ones
who bore these names — and to the work of
our future — ending AIDS.

The Memorial is housed at
www.UncommonHope.org

Please visit the Memorial in its current form
and join the endeavor by remembering
your own losses and submitting their names.

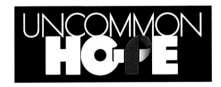

Alvin
Andrew
Bob
Bobby
Chris
Chuck
Dallas
Dana
David
Deacon Marty
Den
Edwin
Frank
Gary
Gerry
Henry
Ja
Jacqueline
Jeff
Jennifer
Jerry
Jim
John
Ken
Kevin
Kris
Lee
Lisa
Mark
Markie
Martin
Michael
P.B.
Patrick
Paul
Randy
Ray
Ricky
Rob
Ron
Scott
Shelby
Sonny
Steve
TC
Tim
Toby
Tony

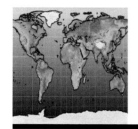

CHAPTER 1

"A people without the knowledge of their past history, origin and culture is like a tree without roots."

Marcus Garvey *1887-1940*

"I was ordained in 1996 and served as volunteer clergy on staff at Metropolitan Community Church of San Francisco for the next 10 years, but I was never to know the experience of AIDS at that church as so many others did. I wasn't there when 500+ people died. I know the history and I know the stories, but I don't know the experience in my body and in my heart the way my colleagues and so many of the congregants do. Sometimes that lack of direct involvement brings up regrets and doubts about my ability to offer the best support to people living with HIV and AIDS. Working on Metropolitan Community Churches' *Uncommon Hope* Curriculum helped me recognize that I can only do what I can do now: learning about the history, taking action today, and reminding myself of the words we used in the HIV Ministry when I was pastoring at Wichita Falls MCC – There is no day but today."

Rev. Lea Brown *Metropolitan Community Church of San Francisco*

Looking Back & Working Forward:
History & Timelines of HIV and AIDS

Overview of Chapter

The work of bringing an end to AIDS requires a global response built on the foundations of individual action, informed decisions, collective commitment and historically-based understanding. A well-informed community with a working knowledge of its historical experience with HIV and AIDS can respond to the changing nature of the pandemic from a place of strength rather than one of crisis.

Every community of faith has a unique experience with HIV and AIDS. The factors informing that experience may include:

- the loss of loved ones,
- activism,
- silence,
- apathy,
- denial, and/or
- previous successful or unsuccessful efforts to build a supportive network.

Though the details of the past are different for various groups and individual group members, it is the collective awareness of our shared history that creates a strong foundation for a powerful and innovative future.

At the end of this chapter, you will find several articles and reference to a listing of resource materials. These documents offer snapshots of AIDS and HIV over time: rather than presenting a complete picture of the past three decades, the materials serve as guideposts to how HIV and AIDS were viewed, discussed and addressed at key moments. You and your group of participants will need to decide how many of the articles to use, what resources to access, and how best to use and incorporate your selections. In our pilot programs, some groups chose to read a number of articles collectively; others opted for individual or sub-group readings with summary reports and feedback to the entire group. Also included at the end of this chapter is a partial transcript of an address delivered by Joshua Love at Lancaster Theological Seminary. You may wish to play the talk (available for viewing on the *Uncommon Hope* DVD, Chapter 2) as a warm-up activity for the group as you begin this unit. Participants can then read the transcript later or simply refer back to the video presentation in their discussions.

The readings will lay the groundwork for beginning to research and create your own community's HIV and AIDS timeline. Generating your own timeline can open powerful insight into *how* and *when* your community of faith has been successful in its public activism and where it has work to do preparing for a more engaged future.

One potential project that might develop from this unit is a display for exhibit in the church or other public space to the congregation and/or the larger community. The project can be extended and made interactive by including a response component (perhaps a book containing recollections, personal stories and blank pages) and encouraging viewers to add their own memories of how the church or community engaged with HIV and AIDS.

AGENDA FOR SESSION

Notes to the Facilitator
Room Set-Up
Full group discussion for the *Uncommon Hope* program works best in a circle if group size permits. If your meeting space will not accommodate such an arrangement, then angled rows from which participants can easily turn to see their peers in other seats will work. It is very important to check on sound and noise levels to ensure that participants will be able to hear presentations as well as each other's comments and feedback. You may wish to break into pairs or small groups for parts of the discussion; if so, plan ahead for any movement of people or furniture. As much as possible, try to anticipate any physical accomodations your participants may need — larger print materials or the services of an ASL or BSL interpreter, for example.

Readings
In order to derive maximum benefit from this session, participants should have access to the articles at the back of this chapter in advance of the meeting time. It is recommended that they read them all if time allows. If not, then have them select several that "grab" their attention. Each article can be copied from this facilitator's guide.

Supplies
This session requires copies of the articles you have selected from the resource section at the end of this chapter. You may also want to have on hand a DVD player with speakers for playback, personal inventory sheets, construction paper, magazines or similar sources for images/illustrations, rulers, crayons, colored markers, scissors and other craft supplies as well as pencils/pens and a notebook including paper suitable for journaling, for each person.

Time requirements
The preferred session length is either 4 hours with a snack or meal break in the middle, or two sessions of 2 hours each separated by approximately two weeks. Once the creation of a timeline is begun, there is often the need to divide participants into groups for a time of discussion and research before their findings can be put into final form. Regardless of the session length you opt for, do plan on short, hourly breaks. If your session does include a meal, assign small group discussion during that extended break. When people are beginning to know each other, some of the most exciting bonding and sharing can take place in the context of eating together.

Introductions and Warm-Up Exercises
Each session of *Uncommon Hope* offers participants the opportunity to explore their own spiritual lives more deeply and to connect more profoundly with others in the group. The process begins at an almost unconscious level when participants first enter the workshop space and becomes overt as individuals share their names a little more formally in the time set for introductions. To further promote the transition from "outside lives" to the special time of group interaction, you should engage the group in a mindfully preparatory exercise at the beginning of each session. Each community may create its own introductory experiences or you may draw from the activities list provided in the Appendix.

The scripts given below are samples intended primarily for first-time facilitators. They can be used "as is" or modified to suit the needs and comfort of the facilitator and/or the group.

Sample Script
Introduction of the Facilitator *(suggested time: 2 minutes)*
Welcome to the first session of *Uncommon Hope.* I am *(Name and Community Affiliation).* The title of the workshop session I will be facilitating today is **Looking Back & Working Forward: The History and Timelines of HIV and AIDS.** My experience with HIV and AIDS is *(Your Story...)* I am committed to participating in ongoing efforts to support people living with HIV and AIDS and to bringing an end to the AIDS pandemic because *(give your reasons.)* I am so glad you have come to add your hearts and voices to this life-changing work.

Introduction of Participants and (Sample) Warm-Up Exercise *(suggested time: 30 seconds to 1 minute per participant for this warm-up exercise; times for the different introductory activities in the Appendix will vary.)*
We will have the opportunity to get to know a lot about one another as we progress through the *Uncommon Hope* curriculum. To get that process started let's take a few minutes to learn each other's names and do a quick a warm-up exercise. Please tell the group your name, the place you call home, and respond to the prompt: "One of my life heroes is ___ because ___." in less than a minute. We will begin with a volunteer and then we can go around the circle. *Ask for a volunteer.*

INTRODUCTION TO SESSION 1
*The Facilitator should read the guidelines section to the group
and have these posted around the room if possible*

Group Guidelines
Exploring the unique and diverse experiences of community in a group context challenges us to be open to new ways of thinking. Old ideas and feelings may be triggered, unexpected disagreements may arise, and individuals in the discourse may hear information in a manner that is distinctly their own. Strive to maintain your awareness that each person brings a singular context (history, social norms, belief systems, and needs) to the dialogue.

The following guidelines have been adapted from the work of VISIONS, Inc. They have encouraged better listening skills in teachers, preachers, and students of all ages, races, social classes, and spiritual backgrounds; and they will be of vital importance to us as we work in community to tear down the walls that separate us and build up the hope for a future in which the wide range of human experience is honored with respect and dignity.

Try On: New Ideas, Content, and Process
This course will invite us to be creative and open to new learning, to "try on" some new ideas, processes, and content. Bear in mind that by consenting to experiment with new points of view, you're not abandoning your current beliefs — you may well choose to pick them back up again later — but see if for the time we gather in this study, you might explore some new

ways of behaving and belonging. Just like our bodies change over time, so do our minds, emotions, and spirits. This guideline will allow us to explore ideas and ways of being in community that, along with our ever-evolving experiences, may better fit our dynamic sense of self in the world.

It Is OK to Disagree: It Is Not OK to Shame, Blame, or Attack...Others or Ourselves
As we share passionately held beliefs, explore our deepest emotions and investigate our social context, disagreements and differences of opinion are likely to surface. A conscious awareness that we are "trying on" new ideas which may not always fit can be a great first step toward conflict resolution. The next step is to acknowledge that disagreeing is an authentic and acceptable reaction at certain points of the journey. Be mindful that a respectful process of disagreement does not involve shaming, blaming, or attacking anyone, ourselves included, for the expression of different feelings, experiences or ideas.

Practice Self-Focus
This guideline will allow us to learn and explore our experience of community from our various, unique perspectives. Part 1 of practicing self-focus is to employ the simple but powerful tool of the "I statement": I feel happy when... vs. People feel happy when... Secondly, let's utilize increased self-awareness to notice our own thoughts and feelings as we listen to each other. Instead of mentally rehearsing comments and rebuttals to the sharing of other group members, we can use this tool to receive whatever is being shared more completely and to appreciate its impact more fully.

Practice "Both/And" Thinking
Western culture encourages an individualistic way of exploring ideas, and places great value on being "right" and having the correct answer or approach in any given situation. As a consequence, most of us have learned to perceive relationships and community from the mindset of "either/or"—right or wrong, good or bad. Shifting to a "both/and" viewpoint will allow each of us to explore our group process from a variety of perspectives and learn in a rich context without needing to feel compromised or wrong. The practical application of this guideline is simple and straightforward; just replace the word "but" in a sentence with the word "and". For example: I believe that Christianity is the best spiritual path for me, **and** I accept that other people's self-determined best pathways will be different.

Take Responsibility for Your Own Learning
As adults, we tend to approach learning, particularly in a group environment, quite differently from the way we did when we were children or adolescents. Simply put "life happens" and we know ourselves well enough to know when we have reached our limits. There are times when each of us needs to take an intentional break, handle an assignment in a different way, or use a personal "course correction" to reach our goals. This journey is intended to empower the best aspects of group process and self-awareness, so if you need to ask for support or make a shift to gain maximum benefit, don't wait for the facilitator(s) to "figure it out." Ask for what you need. Your ownership and expression of your unique learning style will add value to your experience and that of the group. Find a person or persons with whom to share your strategies and create accountability to support your own continued learning.

Be Aware of the Difference between Intent and Impact

When engaging in a communal learning process it is incredibly valuable to consider the difference between intent and impact. Comments and feedback can be offered with the clearest of intentions and still be experienced by others in ways that have markedly negative impacts. There is no perfect failsafe to prevent this from happening; however, maintaining an awareness of intent and impact can lessen negative experiences and reduce conflicts. To implement this guideline, slow down, return to self-focus, and assume best intent on the part of your peers before engaging in reactions that might blame, shame, or attack.

In the moment, from a place of best intent and self-focus, each of us can consider the impact of another's comments and can then communicate gently when a negative experience occurs. A couple of great words to help with this process are "Ouch" and "Oops." The first allows us to tell others that their impact on us has been painful; the second lets us say, "I'm sorry," if we fear our comments may have landed with negative impact. Either word can be used without diverting the conversation or requiring lengthy explanations.

Maintain Confidentiality About Personal Sharing

This learning experience will afford us the opportunities to share very personal experiences, memories, and insights. In order to cultivate a culture of safety and mutual respect, we will need to have a common understanding of the standard we'll apply to information that is shared within the group. A general rule of thumb for whether or not it is appropriate to discuss shared personal stories outside of the group setting can be summed up as follows: if you didn't bring it in to the room with you, then don't take it out of the room with you. Gossip, whether intentional or accidental, can be corrosive to the group's integrity, so let us agree to avoid, as best we can, retelling other people's stories or experiences without their explicit permission.

Taking consciousness of confidentiality one step further can help us to establish healthy boundaries and positive standards for spiritual care. When people share their personal stories, we can demonstrate respect for their privacy by securing their permission before pursuing further discussion with them outside of the group process. Whether we're at lunch or in church or on the phone, we can honor this group's sacred, safe space by not reentering discussions begun "on the inside" without permission to do so. Remember, of course, that when you ask another person for permission to continue a conversation, "no" and "not now" are valid responses and must be honored.

The original contents of the guidelines were developed by VISIONS, Inc. and are respectfully used with permission of VISIONS, Inc. (http://www.visions-inc.org/)

SMALL GROUP EXERCISE 1

Select one or two of the articles at the end of the chapter for each small group to read. When they've accomplished the reading, ask them to consider the following items and discuss their responses with each other.

Things to Think About and Questions for Reflection
Describe and discuss your reactions to the articles that your group read.

What emotions do these looks at HIV and AIDS through the years bring up for you?

What are your earliest memories of public information about HIV and AIDS?

When did you first hear about HIV and AIDS? Do you remember the year?

At what point were you able to find useful and helpful information about HIV and AIDS in your communities?

Do you know when your local newspapers began reporting on HIV and AIDS?

When was the first AIDS Service Organization (ASO) created in your community?

What was the first response by your local church (or hospital or other organization) to HIV and AIDS?

Which of the recommendations/actions described in the articles you read might you or your organization somehow implement or incorporate?

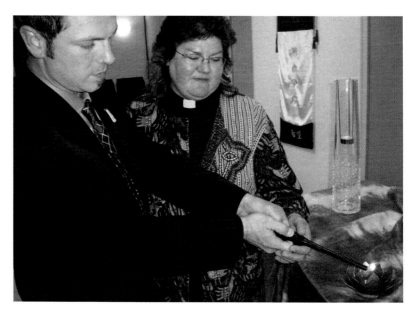

Rev. Kharma Amos and Joshua L. Love prepare the altar for World AIDS Day 2007 at MCC Northern Virginia.

Develop an HIV and AIDS Timeline for viewing or presentation at your church (or other organization). Your timeline could take any number of forms. For example, your group might produce a poster series that takes the pandemic and breaks it out into accessible timeframes, or you might create a book with articles that are relevant to your local community and the national HIV and AIDS timelines. A sample of an HIV/AIDS Timeline is included in this book (page 13).

CLOSING MEDITATION/POEM/PRAYER/RITUAL/SONG

Note to the Facilitator
This can be created by the participants or drawn from any resource that is compatible with the faith traditions represented in the group.

It is night.

The night is for stillness.
Let us be still in the presence of God.

It is night after a long day.
What has been done has been done; what has not been done has not been done; let it be.

From a longer prayer in
A New Zealand Prayer Book/He Karakia Mihinare o Aotearoa, *authorized by General Synod on 26 May 1988 pursuant to the 1928 Church of England Empowering Act procedures, for use in the Church of the Province of New Zealand, in terms of the Canons of the General Synod.*

God gives power to the faint, and strengthens the powerless...God shall renew their strength, they shall mount up with wings like eagles, they shall run and not be weary, they shall walk and not faint.

Isaiah 40:29-31

Fear is not the enemy unless we allow it to become that. We could welcome our fear for the opportunity it brings us to develop fearlessness.

Carolyn Rose Gimian from "Smile at Fear" in Shambhala Sun, *March 2009*

RESOURCES AND ARTICLES

Note to the Facilitator

In addition to the reprinted articles and lecture transcription which follow, there are useful resource materials listed in the Bibliography & Suggested Readings at the back of this book. The identification and compilation of resources for this unit is an ongoing process. As that body of support materials grows, and in particular expands to reflect a greater diversity of experience and viewpoints, newly available resources will be posted to the Chapter 1 section of the website *www.UncommonHope.org*.

It should be noted that the articles included here are reprinted as written and some of them include language (and by extension, ideology) that may startle, discomfit or even offend some participants. For example, in 2008 we might speak of a "person living with AIDS" whereas speakers in 1984 would likely have referred to "an AIDS victim." Such usage could have impact on, and prompt discussion within your group(s). Mention is made here so that you, the facilitator, are not caught off guard.

Selections

AIDS: A Pastoral, Ethical Response
by Rev. Ken Martin
1983

AIDS and the Church
by Earl E. Shelp and Ronald H. Sunderland
1985

We Are the Church Alive, the Church with AIDS
by Kittredge Cherry and Rev. Jim Mitulski
1988

Global HIV: Hope and Injustice
by Rev. A. Stephen Pieters
1996

Fractured Faith/Uncommon Hope: AIDS and the Church
by Joshua L. Love
2008

HIV and AIDS - Changing All the Time...Still!
by Joshua L. Love
2008

HIV and AIDS in 2008
by Reverend Nancy L. Wilson
2008

AIDS: A PASTORAL, ETHICAL RESPONSE

by Rev. Ken Martin

This article was first published in the June/July 1983 issue of Journey, *a magazine of the Metropolitan Community Churches General Conference. At the time of publication, Rev. Martin was the pastor at MCC in the Valley in North Hollywood, California (USA).*

First, a very close friend, who is also a clergyperson in UFMCC, called to tell me he had been given a "preliminary diagnosis of AIDS." Less than two weeks later I conducted the funeral service of a 29 year old victim of AIDS. His family chose not to even acknowledge the service. Two days later an active member of our church came into my office to tell me he had AIDS. On Easter Sunday a long time friend, and partner in ministry at Good Shepherd Parish MCC in Chicago, came to me and said, "I just came to say 'good-bye' and tell you 'I love you.'" Three weeks later he was dead of AIDS. I participated in his funeral service at MCCLA.

What do we in UFMCC say in response to this threat and horror called AIDS? In addition to keeping ourselves informed regarding the information from the Center for Disease Control, other research programs, the sensitivity and awareness of medical professionals in our respective areas, and the local and national AIDS support groups within our own communities, should we as a unique and spiritual body begin formulating an equally unique and spiritual response?

I believe the answer is yes. As a people whose every action and decision must be guided by the Good News that God was present in Jesus Christ and continues that presence with us through the Holy Spirit, we must bring the same innovative and creative energy to this issue that we are attempting to bring to so many others with which we are faced.

I would like for the remainder of this article to be seen as nothing more than a beginning. The four points of departure which I shall discuss are, to me, crucial. However, they are in no way exhaustive. I invite other persons within UFMCC to revise and augment them. Seeing this, therefore, as the beginning of a process, I would like to suggest that we internalize and actualize at least the following four awarenesses in our response.

First, we must remain a sex-positive people.

AIDS Victim: "I should have known that God would punish me for having too much fun."

One of the most tragic mistakes we could make would be to become a sex-negative people, even inadvertently. Both in language and attitude we must avoid any indication that AIDS is in any way a "plague" or "punishment" being visited upon us because of our sexuality.

Instead, it is a time for an intense and personal evaluation, on the part of Gay males, of our sexual patterns, and caution and restraint in activities known to put one at increased risk.

Two thousand years of ignorance, fear, guilt, and shame regarding human sexuality (to say nothing of homosexuality) is just beginning to be reversed within Christian thought, writings and practice. I believe that the existence and witness of UFMCC has been an inextricable factor in this reversal. To abdicate that influence now, an influence I believe God has clearly called us to, would constitute sin on our parts.

Second, we must create spiritual support systems for victims, spouses, families and friends.

Spouse of AIDS Victim: "Our friends were afraid to come to the hospital. Toward the end, they wouldn't even come to the house. They didn't even call but I think that was because they felt guilty."

The Ministerial Staff of our church has notified local media and AIDS support groups that we are available for visits and counseling to AIDS victims, spouses and families. One of the most tragic things surrounding this illness is the designation of the AIDS victim as a "contemporary leper." Even professional health workers have expressed their apprehension at dealing with those who have AIDS. I believe our model for ministry here is Francesco Bernadoni, later known as St. Francis of Assisi. Born into a wealthy, aristocratic family, Francis confessed a repugnance and revulsion for lepers. After a profound personal Christian faith commitment, Francis encountered a leper on the road outside Assisi. He dismounted his horse, threw his coat over the leper, kissed him and began to ride away. When he looked back

there was no one there. To his death, Francis believed that he had encountered Christ. (Hebrews 13:2)

For the families and friends of many persons, a diagnosis of AIDS becomes an unprepared-for disclosure of sexual orientation. While responses are most often uninformed and frequently cruel, they are eventually Biblical and spiritual in nature. OPPORTUNITY FOR MINISTRY! Don't miss it.

Third, we must provide financial support for AIDS research.

Dr. Joel Weisman: "How many people have to die before there's an all-out effort?"

Several governmental health officials have now acknowledged that their response to AIDS has been "too little and too late." Some have even acknowledged the homophobic basis for this lack of action. We know that while fewer persons died of Legionnaire's Disease or Toxic Shock Syndrome (which in no way diminishes the severity of these or the appropriateness of response to them) both public concern and research appropriations were much more rapidly forthcoming. Therefore, we must remain persistently active. First, we must continue to insist upon large single grants from public and private sources, and second, we must mobilize every organization and institution within our Gay and Lesbian communities to raise funds.

Fourth, we must seek a standard by which to evaluate our sexual behavior during and after this crisis.

Parishioner to Pastor: "Please tell me what is OK and what's not OK for me to do sexually."

Talking about sex is not easy for most of us. When we try to talk about it in the context of our understanding of Christian responsibility and freedom it usually becomes even more difficult. Even after two years of doctoral study in human sexuality I usually find that I am eventually asked more questions than I am prepared to answer! However, I have been able to settle upon three certainties which are, as of yet, unshakable to me. First, being sexual is good and sex is fun. Second, sex is not just a biological instinct in women and men. It is a gift, a part of our createdness as the children of God. It is not just procreative, it is creative. It is a serious and wonderful part of us, and therefore involves responsibility and must be taken seriously. Third, genital sexuality, i.e. sex acts, are, in and of themselves, morally neutral: they are good or bad/right or wrong/moral or immoral according to the quality of the experience. So, even though it is the right thing I am often asked to do, I refuse to create lists of "dos and don'ts, cans and can'ts, shoulds and should nots, etc." That has been done by almost every denomination and tradition within Christendom. And, the results have never been any too positive for us or many others!

Realizing then that there is no easy answer; is there any scriptural standard for us? Is there a guideline, a test by which we may consistently evaluate our sexual behavior? I believe there is and I believe it is found in Galatians 5:13.

"...you were called, as you know, to liberty; but be careful, or this liberty will provide an opening for self-indulgence. Serve one another, rather, in works of love, since the whole of the Law is summarized in a single command: Love your neighbor as yourself."

Within Christianity, then, the new principle which determines everything — including our sexual behavior — is love. Can our sexual behavior submit to the test of love?

We are free ("at liberty") to acknowledge and explore our sexuality. We are free from graceless moralism, codified sexual ethics, and antiquated myths. We are not free to minimize or disregard our sexuality which is a wonder-full part of ourselves. It has inordinate constructive potential and considerable destructive potential. What we are free to do is love: submit our every action and expression to the test of love.

Perhaps we, more than many, realize that we have been created by love, that we have been sought and called out by Jesus Christ and empowered to live in love. When our actions as sexual beings cannot submit to the test of love we know that God is more concerned about us than what we do. God is more concerned about the estrangement, fear, frustration, anxiety, and especially the loneliness that leads to an unloving sexual encounter than what may happen afterwards.

While I am in no way trying to say that AIDS is the consequence of encounters which cannot submit to the test of love, I am trying to take seriously the preponderance of research which indicates that those who are most at risk are those who are "sexually intimate with many partners." I am also taking the opportunity — which many have expressed as long overdue — to call for a reevaluation of sexual patterning which may characterize a significant portion of the Gay male community.

AIDS, along with its related problems and issues, is a serious concern which is now affecting populations other than just Gay males. The approach I have attempted to outline here is just a beginning for all of us who believe that the Gospel calls us to be present whenever the quality of life is at issue for any person.

article
AIDS AND THE CHURCH

by Earl E. Shelp and Ronald H. Sunderland

The church, however, was noticeably silent. In fact, since 1981 when AIDS was first described, the personal tragedies and social failures associated with the disease appear to have been largely ignored by the church – except for those strident segments that view AIDS as God's retribution on a sinful people.

This silence may imply assent to the view that certain at-risk populations (gay and bisexual men, drug addicts, prostitutes) deserve the disease and the horrible death it portends. Or the silence may indicate a lack of knowledge of the disease and of the opportunities for ministry it generates. Whatever the reason for the shortcoming, AIDS raises basic issues of pastoral and prophetic ministry that involve the church's role in the community as well as its responsibility for society's dispossessed. Whether or not the federal government or other agencies provide resources to meet this crisis and some of the needs of people touched by it, the church itself must respond if it is to reflect in its life the spirit of its Lord who commanded his fellow servants to do for one another what he had done for them.

The Gospel of Luke is noted for its emphasis on Jesus as the humble, loving, compassionate Christ who holds the poor, the outcast and the dispossessed in special regard (see particularly Luke 4:16-30 and 7:18-23). Liberation theologians have developed this theme as the springboard for their theologies. An uncompromising affirmation of the church's ministry to the poor is central to the church's servanthood, they urge, since Jesus came preaching the Good News to the poor, and announcing freedom to the broken victims of human indignities and oppression. God's servants have a special responsibility to act with justice and righteousness, and to speak prophetically in the name of a just, righteous and compassionate God.

The Jewish community could not fathom that the offer and blessing of the end-time would be extended to the despised of society. Yet this was exactly what Jesus proclaimed, drawing on the prophetic understanding of the poor as those who are oppressed, and who, therefore, cannot speak for themselves. The nature of grace and faith revealed in the life and mission of Jesus is demonstrated by his identification with isolated and outcast individuals. The political and religious establishments turn away all too easily from those who are outside the realm of social and religious respectability. Luke's Jesus, however, deliberately turned toward those who had been rejected not only by their community but often by their families. He touched them, ate with them, and announced that they had a place of honor at the heavenly feast.

Jesus never stopped proclaiming that all are equal beneficiaries of God's grace and forgiveness. In fact, he strengthened the proclamation by providing grace and forgiveness through healing, reconciling families and satisfying hunger. In short, Jesus responded compassionately to those broken by life. Often his acts of "pastoral ministry" express God's acceptance and love of those judged unacceptable and unlovable by society, but often Jesus' mere presence beside the dispossessed was itself a manifestation of God's favor toward the powerless.

Luke's Jesus leaves us little room for negotiation, as indicated in the Parable of the Feast (14:15 ff.) in which the invitees state their reasons for declining the invitation to the feast, only to be excluded altogether. Servanthood involves being a sign of the Good News. Our care for others witnesses to our belief that they are also worthy of God's love, and that they can be related to God. Caring not only means that one meets another's immediate needs, but it also calls us to tell the disenfranchised that she or he may become a liberated, loved and loving being.

As is well known, about 73 percent of AIDS patients are homosexual or bisexual men. An additional 17 percent are intravenous drug users. The mainstream of society tends to stigmatize both groups. If their "personal lives" become known, too often they are rejected by family, friends and church, lose employment, and experience other subtle and overt forms of discrimination. And, in the cases of homosexual and bisexual men, the stigma

applies to who they are — a matter about which they have no choice — rather than (or in addition to) what they do — a matter about which they do have a choice.

These injustices are compounded when one is diagnosed as having AIDS or ARC (AIDS-Related Complex). When heterosexual men and women, children, hemophiliacs and people who have received blood transfusions are labeled with AIDS or ARC, they begin to learn what it means to be unjustly isolated and ostracized. Nearly all AIDS or ARC patients have been shunned in some way by a public that fears their disease, objects to their sexuality or disapproves of their conduct. However, in light of Luke's message, the latter two reasons are insufficient to justify Christians' turning away.

Neither should fear of contagion stop Christians from ministering to AIDS patients. The virus associated with AIDS and ARC — *LAV/HTLV III* — is not airborne, and there is no evidence that casual contact with patients results in infection. A person would have to be in contact with an infected person's bodily fluids (blood, excretions, secretions) to be at risk of contracting the virus. Protective precautions (gloves, mask, garments) are usually needed only during a patient's hospitalization or when certain nursing procedures are performed outside of the hospital. It should also be noted that some people who have been infected by the virus for as long as three years have not as yet manifested the disease. This suggests that factors in addition to infection by *LAV/HTLV III* may contribute to the development of AIDS. Adequate instruction and proper precautions, as indicated, should ease, if not totally remove, any fears that might hinder ministry to these people in need.

Some Christians might also be reluctant to minister to AIDS patients out of fear that the social isolation of AIDS victims will be extended to those who befriend them. Colleagues and friends may withdraw, apparently fearing contagion, or because they disapprove of the investment in AIDS patients. Physicians, nurses and others who provide medical care to these patients have experienced this type of rejection. Christians should remember, however, that Jesus did not let the reaction of others deter him from having fellowship with the alienated and "unclean." The course of the disease varies among patients. Part of its insidiousness is its unpredictability.

The single constant is that no patient survives. Medical scientists around the world have moved with remarkable speed to identify *LAV/HTLV III* — a virus that can weaken, even destroy, the body's immune system. Unfortunately, no antiviral agent, vaccine or therapy to restore an immunity system has been found effective. Though physicians are improving their ability to treat symptoms with approved drugs and experimental agents, at best this enables some patients to live longer. At worst, it prolongs their lives so that they only suffer greater indignities and die more distressing deaths.

More than 600 AIDS or ARC patients have been registered in the clinic where we consult. An additional five to ten patients are treated as inpatients, about half of whom die during their hospitalization. Most AIDS patients valiantly try to maintain their independence as long as possible. But as they become too weak to work, as they lose income, medical insurance and possibly living quarters, as they suffer losses of eyesight and mental function and as they face social ostracism, AIDS victims can slip into almost total dependence on family, lovers and friends — who may or may not remain

committed to them. Indeed, the intensity of this terminal disease's physical and emotional toll may provoke the loss of one's total support system.

Out of a desire not to hurt, embarrass or burden them, some homosexual or bisexual patients keep their sexuality and illness from family members. Even when told that a family member is dying, some families have refused to help. And parents and siblings who do not abandon patients frequently go through this trauma without the understanding and support of other family members and friends, or of their congregations, choosing, for whatever reason or reasons, to bear this burden privately. Their concern for secrecy may extend to requests that death certificates not reveal AIDS as a cause of death.

The personal tragedies, unmet needs and social failures extend far beyond those indicated here. Instead of compassion, the overwhelming public and political response to AIDS has been fear and callousness. For example, some health-care personnel and hospitals in the Houston area have refused to provide services, and nursing homes have closed their doors to AIDS patients. On August 26 the state of Texas, on the basis of a 9-7 decision of the Fifth U.S. Circuit Court of Appeals, reinstated a law against homosexual activity; it appears that that decision may in part have been influenced by an AIDS-induced backlash. And while Health and Human Services Secretary Margaret Heckler has termed AIDS the number-one priority of the public health service, the Reagan administration has consistently requested relatively small sums to combat the disease.

AIDS has already taken the lives of more than 6,000 people. Tens — perhaps hundreds — of thousands of people from every walk of life will die before treatments are found either to inhibit the disease's progress or to cure it. In the interval, its physical and social ramifications will escalate the suffering of its victims.

The church and individual Christians can help to alleviate the suffering associated with AIDS — particularly in urban areas, where nearly all AIDS patients either reside or go for treatment. The people of God need to remember that the neighbor whom Jesus instructed his disciples to love excludes no one. Congregations' ministries to sick people and to their families ought not to neglect people with AIDS and their natural or chosen families.

Patients with AIDS can become very weak, either quickly or gradually. Often they do not have enough energy to make the almost daily visits to their physicians that are necessary, or to provide for themselves at home. They could benefit greatly by volunteer help: people to shop for them, do light housekeeping tasks, prepare or deliver simple meals, and visit or phone to check on them. The decline in strength is often paralleled by a deterioration of finances. Whatever assets the victim may have are liquidated to pay for medical care. Cars become an unaffordable luxury, so transportation to the clinic becomes a vital need. Financial assistance to purchase everyday needs may be helpful. AIDS patients are often alone, with no one to hear their fears, frustrations and anxieties, or to engage in pleasant conversation. Being a friend to patients can contribute to the quality of their remaining life.

Distant family members who visit the AIDS patient may not be able (or may not want) to stay in the patient's residence. Commercial housing for days or weeks can be a heavy financial burden on top of the emotional stress of watching a loved one die. Providing a bed, transportation, meals and emotional support to these people would be valuable services that Christians could extend. And at the death of the patient, the family may need assistance in making arrangements with a local mortician and in attending to other legal matters.

Finally, pastors could remind parishioners that reconciliation is a key element of the gospel. Reconciliation in the context of AIDS could take place, for example, between the church and homosexuals where they are estranged. Similarly, reconciliation between families and a separated family member could be promoted. Too often family members rush in when the patient is near death trying to affirm their continuing love. Though these reunions should be celebrated, they usually occur so late that the precious opportunities for each to enjoy the other's gifts are few or lost altogether.

AIDS sets before the church an opportunity to reflect on its identity and its mission. For the church to ignore the needs that cluster around AIDS, to fail to express itself redemptively, and to abandon a group of people who have almost no one to cry out in their behalf for justice and mercy, would constitute a failure in Christian discipleship.

WE ARE THE CHURCH ALIVE, THE CHURCH WITH AIDS

by Kittredge Cherry and Rev. Jim Mitulski

Copyright ©1988 by the Christian Century. *Reprinted by permission from the Jan. 27, 1988, issue of the* Christian Century. *At the time of publication, Ms. Cherry was a student minister and women's programming coordinator at Metropolitan Community Church of San Francisco, Rev. Mitulski was pastor of the church, and both were seminarians at Pacific School of Religion in Berkeley, California (USA).*

"Heaven has as much to do with life before death as with life after death." Steven Clover was able to voice that vision in the last months before he died of AIDS, as his body fought off rare forms of cancer, pneumonia and other disease. Once dapper and golden-haired, he was the essence of a refined gentleman, the sort who might own a couple of jewelry stores in Boston — which he did. He also served as an assistant pastor of a black church, Union Baptist Church in Cambridge. He left all that behind in August 1986 to attend Pacific School of Religion in Berkeley and Metropolitan Community Church of San Francisco (MCC-SF), a predominantly white church in a denomination that ministers to the lesbian and gay community.

In October of that year he was diagnosed with AIDS, and as Christmas approached he was hospitalized. Thirty children from a black Baptist church in San Francisco showed up at the hospital to sing carols for Clover and other people with AIDS (commonly referred to as PWAs.) In the ensuing months he was able to bring together the congregations of Double Rock Baptist Church, which condemns homosexuality as a sin, and MCC-SF, which preaches that homosexuality is a gift from God.

These seemingly irreconcilable churches sponsored events together, including a gospel music concert that raised more than $1,000 for the San Francisco AIDS Foundation Food Bank in July 1987. Clover died a month later.

Clover's church is our church, MCC-SF, which is encircled by San Francisco's biggest gay and lesbian neighborhood. And in many ways, Clover's story is our story. What he and others have experienced individually, we have undergone and still undergo as an institution. We believe that our drama is having an impact on the larger body of the whole Christian community, especially churches whose members include parents, relatives and friends of PWAs.

Currently, we know of 30 congregants who have AIDS, and the number threatens to keep rising. About two-thirds of the men in the congregation are "antibody positive," a sign that they have been in contact with the AIDS virus. Every week our worship service attracts at least one person who was just diagnosed. Death also attends weekly — the death of a member or a member's friend. Moreover, we perform several memorial services each month for people with AIDS who have never set foot in our church. Their friends and relatives, who come from churches all across America, turn to us because they know we will welcome them, honor gay relationships, and provide acceptance that they cannot expect from most mainline churches.

Just as our members with AIDS suffer discrimination in housing, employment and medical care, our church suffers anti-AIDS discrimination. For example, a Roman Catholic retreat center said we could not use its facility unless we informed other groups that people with AIDS would be there. We regard this as denying us equal access. For the retreat center, the bottom line was the presence of PWAs in our group. "And what about the bathrooms?" the center coordinator persisted, revealing her ignorance of how AIDS is spread.

We have come to understand ourselves as a church with AIDS. This doesn't mean that our church will soon be dead and gone. No, in fact it means that we live more deeply. The whole gay male community is undergoing a parallel transformation. A lifestyle characterized by carefree promiscuity has given way to dating and friendship. Many people are seeking intimacy and spirituality, which has had the effect of a revival. Thus, despite the deaths of many members, our membership has actually grown by a third in the past year.

The Universal Fellowship of Metropolitan Community Churches (UFMCC) was founded in Los Angeles in 1968 by Troy Perry, a former Pentecostal minister who aimed to spread the new gospel that God loves gays and lesbians. "All we had time to do was to celebrate and to grow," recalled Howard Wells, who founded MCC-SF in 1969. Grow we did: today there are more than 30,000 MCC members in more than 200 churches worldwide. But our innocent sense of celebration has died of AIDS. Wells,

himself a PWA, says we now live with the end in sight, a state, he calls "eschatological living."

"The specter of AIDS catapults us into accelerated spiritual growth — or toward early death — and it all depends on the model of eschatological living we choose to follow," he said. On good days, being a church with AIDS helps us to see how fragile and important every moment is. We rediscover images — such as heaven — that we used to dismiss as anachronistic or overly sentimental. We claim for ourselves the model known in Scripture as "the realm of God," which Wells defines "an alternative way of living."

It's not easy. Institutionally, we suffer the stages of grief on a grand scale, ricocheting through denial, anger, bargaining, depression and acceptance. Long-range planning is difficult for the church, just as it is for people with AIDS, who are overwhelmed by having to make plans about wills, medical care and finances. Yet never has planning been more crucial. Promoting church growth feels almost macabre, but without it we cannot meet the challenges ahead.

Sunday worship is marked by tears, laughter and unforgettable singing. One of our favorite hymns was written by UFMCC members Jack St. John and David Pelletier in 1980, before we were aware of AIDS: "We are the church alive, the body must be healed; where strife has bruised and battered us, God's wholeness is revealed." Like Clover, we find that our struggle with AIDS has brought us insights into what it means to build heaven into our everyday lives, to try to realize the realm of heaven here and now.

Our most intimate, intense worship service is the monthly AIDS healing service, at which 15 to 20 people affected by AIDS request and receive laying-on-of-hands prayer from each other. To listen to their stories is to enter into the enormity that is AIDS: a doctor sobs over his inability to heal his best friend; someone who recently tested antibody-positive confesses that his anger has separated him from his friends and his God; a withered man prays simply for an appetite; another person with AIDS proudly proclaims he is "living with AIDS, not dying of it;" a nurse who has accidentally jabbed herself with an AIDS contaminated needle says she feels numb now that ten of her co-workers have died of AIDS. We also hold special services, such as AIDS prayer vigils and the blessing of banners for the NAMES Project quilt that was part of the Lesbian and Gay Rights March on Washington last October. The quilt will be touring 25 U.S. cities later this year.

In a sense, all of our worship services are AIDS healing services. Every Sunday we provide a gay-affirming environment where scripture is related to lesbian and gay experience and same-sex pairs can receive, as a couple, communion and laying-on-of-hands prayer. Our very existence challenges the often-held Christian position that AIDS is God's punishment for the sin of homosexuality, a position that breeds a self-hatred that many of us still struggle to overcome. Recently a young man confessed to the pastor before church that, under parental pressure he had vowed sexual abstinence if God would cure him of AIDS — a typical response and one that reveals the heart of gay self-hatred.

Community Prayer is the phase of Sunday worship when the impact of AIDS is most tangible. We join hands and share words and phrases that crystallize our concerns and joys. Every month we hear more petitions for "my friend who was just diagnosed" or "my lover in the hospital" or "more government funding for AIDS research" or "help with my diagnosis."

Peer support groups provide a spiritual context for people to discuss what they have in common — in this case, a life-threatening illness, or being antibody positive or being a caregiver to a person with AIDS. In addition to these groups that are obviously related to AIDS, our men's retreats and Men Together discussion/ worship series approach the subject indirectly by encouraging men to make and deepen friendships away from bars, the traditional gay male meeting ground. All of these become opportunities for dealing with AIDS-related grief. For example, at the spring 1987 retreat, men wrote, read and discussed their experiences of touching other men. One of the readings discussed was this:

Scott and I spent hard and precious times together from the time he was diagnosed with AIDS in 1983 until he died in 1984. I was at work one day — my great escape from the illness was work — when I suddenly felt the need to be at home… I lay with Scott, all the while telling him how much I loved him. I mentioned every person I could think of and made sure he heard that they loved him as well. Scott's labored breathing continued with long lapses between breaths. Each lapse, I thought, would be his last. At 4:42, Scott's breathing stopped and never began again. I held him in my arms and softly told him again and again how precious he was. We spent 45 minutes alone, with Scott in my arms for the last time. His body grew cold before I was finally able to release my hold of him. That most precious touch was to be our last.

People turn to us for counseling at every stage of the AIDS crisis. Most of this is handled by clergy with support from student clergy and the AIDS Ministry Team. Touching is one of the most important ingredients in all AIDS counseling. Although AIDS cannot be spread through casual contact, people with AIDS tend to be treated as untouchables, which adds to their pain.

A congregant's first AIDS-related counseling often revolves around being tested for AIDS antibodies; a positive result means people can transmit the AIDS virus and may develop AIDS themselves. Just deciding to take the test is excruciating. Even those who imagined they were prepared to face a positive result are often devastated by feelings of grief, guilt and betrayal when the verdict is presented.

AIDS-related counseling also means providing home and hospital visitation, funerals, memorial services and bereavement support. An unforgettable example occurred in summer 1987 when one of us visited an AIDS hospice to take communion to a member, his parents visiting from the East Coast and a few close friends. The man, obviously near death, urged everyone to pray not just for him but for their own needs — a reversal of the angry response he expressed earlier in his illness. "I can see heaven," he told them. "It's a beautiful place, the place you've always wanted to go to, and anyone who wants to can go there." The boundaries of heaven and earth seemed to shift that afternoon, so that they no longer corresponded to birth and death; it felt possible to reach into the skies and tug heaven into the present. Death became "a foretaste of the feast to come."

The man died a few hours later. His mother spoke at his memorial service, with tears in her eyes: "He was the best son a mother could ever have." But she and her husband dreaded going back to their home church, being reluctant to tell anyone in their United Methodist congregation that their son had died of AIDS. They didn't think anyone there would understand.

Another set of parents, also United Methodists, asked one of us to come to their son's hospital bedside to join them in prayer. There the mother asked, "Why are people so mean?" She was referring to unsympathetic church members back home. The next question was even harder: was it OK to pray for their comatose son to die soon? The whole church is coming to see that physical death is not necessarily something to avoid; it can even mean healing.

MCC-SF also strives to educate people outside the gay and lesbian community about AIDS, through letter-writing campaigns, public presentations and workshops on AIDS, which have been given in a variety of settings, including the San Francisco AIDS Interfaith Conference, the United Methodist Consultation on AIDS Ministries, the Presbyterian Ministers Association, and Pacific School of Religion's AIDS Awareness Week. In addition, MCC-SF members enrolled at Pacific School of Religion continually pressure the seminary to live up to its policy of fair treatment for students with AIDS. Joint activities with Double Rock Baptist Church have been educational, too. While we have confronted our racism, the Baptists have had to surmount unfounded fears about catching AIDS. One Double Rock usher described holding hands with gay people during prayer time as "the most growing I have ever done."

In our church, AIDS has also brought reconciliation between the sexes, a rift that has been especially deep between lesbians and gay men. Like other women, lesbians face economic disadvantages. But in the case of lesbians, their resulting anger at men is untempered by romantic involvement with the opposite sex. Most lesbian feminists feel it is a waste of energy to spend it in the traditional female role of helping men, their oppressors. However, that feeling doesn't prevail in our church. When the topic of lesbians ministering to men with AIDS came up during a reception the women of our church held for Karen Ziegler, pastor of the Metropolitan Community Church in New York, Ziegler responded this way: "I don't feel like I'm sacrificing – I receive energy by ministering to men with AIDS." She told us "some men I love very much – my friends David and Tim – began to die of AIDS. I had the experience of coming closer than I ever had come to a man before. David and then Tim opened a door to their souls in a way that I had never experienced before and my heart has been opened in a way it never was before, too. We're all experiencing that transformation together."

We have also connected with Congregation Sha'ar Zahav, a Reform synagogue with a lesbian and gay congregation, located a few blocks from our church. Together we sponsored a reading by award-winning lesbian poet Adrienne Rich. That evening Rich told us, "Lesbians and gay men have confronted mortality. We have mourned our friends and lovers together and we have stitched an extraordinary quilt of memory together . . . I think that the coming together of Jewish and Christian, lesbian and gay and straight congregants is an important part of this. I also think that the coming together those of us who are non-congregants with you is very important."

Making this kind of connection – between Jew and Christian, female and male, gay and straight, black and white, parent and child – is what eschatological living is all about. With the end in sight, we do more to savor and value life, including the people we once viewed as hopelessly different from ourselves. As a church with AIDS, we try to embody eschatological living. AIDS is killing us at the same time that it heals us.

This must be the vision Steven Clover was talking about when he told us, "Heaven has as much to do with life before death as with life after death."

And it must be the vision Rich meant to convey when she wrote the poem that has become a kind of creed for our church:

> My heart is moved by all I cannot save:
>   so much has been destroyed
> I have to cast my lot with those
>   who age after age, perversely,
> with no extraordinary power,
>   reconstitute the world.

This must be what Jesus meant when he said, "Behold, the kingdom of God is in the midst of you."

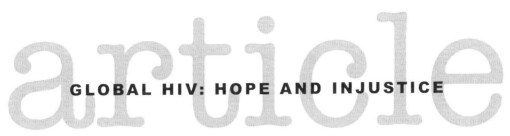

GLOBAL HIV: HOPE AND INJUSTICE

by Rev. A. Stephen Pieters

This essay was written in July of 1996 and appeared as Spirituality Column #16 on the website The Body: The Complete HIV/AIDS Resource (www.thebody.com/content/art5913.html). When the column was written, Rev. Pieters was the Director of AIDS Ministry for Metropolitan Community Churches worldwide.

I had bittersweet feelings as I returned from the XI International HIV/AIDS Conference in Vancouver. On the one hand, I witnessed a prayer being answered. I realized a mission fulfilled.

"Your mission," my doctor told me after my AIDS diagnosis in 1984, "is to stay alive long enough for us to find a way to make the virus manageable, to make it stop destroying the immune system." And I have lived to see that day. Many of us have lived to see that day. Triple combination therapies are working to bring HIV under control, allowing the immune system to restore to near normal levels.

On the other hand, people are still dying, and only 10% of the persons infected with HIV around the world will benefit from these advances, primarily because of economic inequities. Most people with HIV in the world will not be able to access the drugs that can make the infection "chronic and manageable" because they, or their government, will not be able to afford the $15 - 30,000 a year it will cost, in drugs alone, to keep each person with HIV alive. It bears repeating: only 10% of the people infected with HIV in the world will be able to be treated for HIV infection. For the other 90%, the infection will still rapidly progress to AIDS

and death. Most of the people with HIV in the world live in countries where aspirin is hard to access, let alone Crixivan.

HIV further illuminates all the justice issues of our globe: the widening gulf between the "have's" and "have not's" between rich and poor, between developed and developing countries, between men and women.

For me, this conference could have been called, "Global HIV: Hope and Injustice." There are concrete reasons to have hope, and there are real reasons to be angry. There was genuinely good news, finally! And there was too much bad news, still.

On the good news side, researchers announced the resounding success of triple drug "cocktails," combining two antivirals and a protease inhibitor (PI). In 90% of patients tested over six months, viral load has dropped to undetectable levels, and CD4 counts have risen to normal levels. This means that if you take these drugs with great discipline and compliance, you can live with HIV in your body for many, many years with no destruction of the immune system. It was noted again and again, that these are preliminary results, and long term effectiveness has not been established.

My eyes overflowed with tears as I realized that for many sisters and brothers, we are actually, really, honestly going to live normal life spans. I even heard Larry Kramer on the news speak optimistically about HIV for the first time.

And there are countries where HIV education and prevention is working. In countries where frank sex education is allowed, the rate of transmission and the percentage of adults who are infected are as low as in Denmark, with 0.1% of its adult population living with HIV, contrasted with Uganda, where 50% of all adults live and die with HIV. Thailand, Pakistan, Australia and Brazil were all cited as countries where successful risk reduction education has happened, and rates are actually declining in some populations in those countries.

On the flip side, the inaccessibility of treatments is just one injustice. In most of the world, HIV is a "family disease," and there are increasing hordes of uninfected orphaned children, who have lost not only their parents, but all their brothers and sisters. There are few, if any, provisions for these orphans, and they suffer the stigma of being known as "AIDS orphans." Not enough is being done to help them.

In Zambia, one out of five women are infected with HIV before they reach the age of 20. Girls leave their birth families at puberty, and "sugar daddies" adopt them, give them HIV, then throw them out, blaming them for bringing HIV into the house. It can take 3 days to see a doctor, if you live where there are doctors. The woman who gave this particular report thanked the conference for the scholarship which brought her to Vancouver, but demonstrated the economic inequities of this world by pointing out that the registration (around $1,000) would pay her rent for three years, and the plane fare (one can only guess how much that was) would feed her five children into adulthood.

A man from India told me that the government there is not motivated to do prevention education, because they see HIV as the answer to their population problem. Indeed, the country with the most persons with HIV in the world today is India. And even efforts that have been made have had little impact, because Indian men consider homosex to be "mischief" rather than sex, so why should they worry about STD's like HIV? Sexual activity with men is not sex. So how could someone get a sexually transmitted disease? And why would their wives or children be at risk from their "mischief"?

Several speakers addressed the urgent need to empower women to control their own bodies, to be able to protect themselves from HIV and other STD's. We were told that the technology will be in place by the year 2000 for women to be able to protect themselves without their partners' knowledge, and still allow for conception, by using microbicides. The female condom is already available in many areas, of course. Indeed, the "Reality Condom" booth was a very popular exhibit at the conference.

The female condom can also be used by gay men to protect ourselves during anal intercourse, although the FDA will not allow the testing necessary to license it for that use, or even to issue instructions. I asked the exhibitor about this, and she said the FDA wouldn't allow them to do testing for use in anal sex, and then she reached under the table and handed me a booklet with fully illustrated instructions.

The U.S. came under fire for a number of injustices that our government perpetrates. For example, numerous speakers read a litany of some of the countries who will not allow HIV positive travelers to enter their borders: Russia, Iran, Iraq, Saudi Arabia, and the United States. It was chilling to hear my country included with the others who have restrictive immigration laws.

The U.S. was also repeatedly chastised for our failures in HIV prevention efforts. It has been clearly demonstrated in countries like Pakistan, Thailand, Australia, and Brazil that regular, blunt and frank education on reducing risk in sexual activity reduces STD and HIV transmission rates. Furthermore, there is now proof that needle exchange programs work in dramatically reducing transmission rates, with no increase in drug use. But the U.S. government continues to deny the reality of these studies, and so our transmission rate continues to climb.

It's clear that we've turned a corner in treating HIV, and yet there are so many who didn't live to see it happen. I have to qualify every shred of hope now with the reality of the justice issues, the access issues, and the grief issues. I can't get away from it after being at this conference. At the same time that I was crying with joy because I lived to hear the announcement I prayed for, I cried with grief for Fitz, and John, and George, and Nancy, and Linda, and Herbert, and Ron, and on and on, because they didn't.

As if to remind me that we cannot be complacent with the good news, I got back just in time for the deaths of three important people in my life. One of them was Connie Norman, who died July 14. She was a transgendered AIDS diva/warrior, with an angry column ("Tribal Writes") in a popular gay paper in Southern California (Update), and an angry radio talk show. She was a leader of ACT UP LA, and was involved in most everything that went down politically around AIDS in LA since the beginning. I remember being on some commissions with her back in the mid-80's, and being quite in awe. She always had a kind of contempt for me... I just wasn't angry enough.

Then she came to live at the hospice, and I became her chaplain. She began to see my function in life, and she helped me to understand the importance of my own rage about AIDS.

When she died right after the AIDS Conference, it was almost as if there was a transfer of anger from her to me, that I hope I can use positively. I've heard the news I've been waiting to hear for years, and it doesn't bring back all the people this virus has already murdered. It sure didn't do Connie any good. These new advances do not correct the human rights violations that are being perpetrated against women, and the poor, and the sick. The new drug cocktails won't save the lives of more than 1 in 10 of those who have the virus. They don't empower women to control their bodies and their lives. They don't prevent pharmaceutical bureaucrats from making huge fortunes by saving the lives of the rich, and damning whole families of poor people to death.

Yes, it's become chronic and manageable for those of us privileged enough to be in the top ten percentile (and there are plenty of folks with HIV in the U.S. who will not be in that top percentile) but what good does it do when it is still spreading like wildfire, and it will still kill 90% of the people it infects? We've got to eradicate the virus, or it will continue to mow down the population by the millions.

So what do we do? We take action. Hopelessness feeds on helplessness. Hope comes alive when we start doing something. And we must live with hope as we work for justice. We will create hope for ourselves and for all those affected and infected when we take the actions necessary to bring justice to this pandemic.

Every person of faith is called to address justice issues. As Christians, Jesus clearly calls us to demand justice. Demand repeal of the restrictive immigration laws in the U.S. and other countries.

Demand that governments worldwide empower women to control their own STD prevention. Demand that governments worldwide heavily tax the pharmaceutical companies on their profits, to begin to pay for drug access in poor countries. Demand that your government support and fund more effective prevention education. We must continue to educate and to motivate everyone we can to protect themselves from further infections. We must continue to care for the sick and dying.

If you're at risk for HIV, get tested. It can be treated now.

If you're infected, follow your doctor's orders religiously! Your success with these drugs has a direct relationship with how well you follow the instructions on the bottle.

Thank God we've found a way to control HIV. At last, we have really good news from the medical world.

At the same time, we cannot forget that HIV/ AIDS throws a spotlight on all the injustices of this world. For 9 out of 10 persons with HIV in the world, being infected with HIV still has a pretty hopeless outlook.

And that's why we have to take action. That's where we'll find hope. That's where we'll find God.

FRACTURED FAITH/UNCOMMON HOPE: AIDS AND THE CHURCH

by Joshua L. Love (transcribed)

In 2008, Joshua L. Love, Director of the Metropolitan Community Churches Global HIV/AIDS Ministry, delivered the Gregory Lecture on the theme of HIV/AIDS and the Church at Lancaster Theological Seminary. A partial transcript of Love's talk is printed below; the lecture itself was taped and is included on the resource DVD which accompanies the Uncommon Hope *curriculum. (Visit* www.uncommonhope.org *for information about acquiring the DVD.)*

Good Morning.

I want to thank you first of all because this is the prettiest space I've gotten to speak in two and a half years. So, as someone who appreciates the aesthetics as well as the content, I am very grateful to be able to be at such a beautiful place.

We have a lot to do in very little time. I am going to ask you this morning to do a few things and some we will have an opportunity to warm up to and some I am just going to launch into, as well.

First of all, I want you to just look around at the room at the people that are here.

I don't know about you, but I am encouraged to be here engaging in an honest discourse with people who come from different ages, different backgrounds, different ethnic and cultural backgrounds and different racial experiences, different gender identities and expressions.

I am encouraged by that. I am also always disappointed to note that there are empty seats — empty seats which both represent those people who are not ready to engage in this dialogue with us — empty seats which we must acknowledge are the lost lives that AIDS and HIV have taken from us and empty seats who are the people who are lost in their own fear, bigotry and prejudice and cannot bring themselves to ask internal or external questions which would be necessary to be here today.

I am encouraged that you are here and I am encouraged that we are going to have a day that is about telling the truth — the hard truth — the easy truth — and the truth that comes when hope is brought into a conversation that is otherwise incredibly difficult.

The combined weight of our struggles to survive, and overwhelming losses, the combined weight of it all. We still do not have a cure! Is everyone aware of this? I go places sometimes where people do not know. The improvement in medications is not a cure for AIDS. We still do not have one!

See, I am thrilled that we are here today where we can tell the truth about that, because I actually believe we are capable of miracles together...actual, real miracles!

My theology includes a belief that the miracle stories are happening today as much as they were happening when written. It does not matter to me if the Bible is a historical document, it matters to me that in our hearts we hold a place for miracles. So today is a day of miracles and today is a day of healing.

On a personal note, in 1988 AIDS entered into my life. Like many of you, I am sure that I had heard a news article or I had seen someone use the word somewhere. In 1988, my uncle Patrick, a man who had been absent from my life for most of my childhood, returned to Abilene, Texas (where I grew up) to his Church of Christ (and not the United Church of Christ — there is a difference in case you did not know) — to his Church of Christ, conservative evangelical Christian family because he had nowhere else to go. He had lost his job. He was losing what benefits he had left, and he needed a place to die.

You see, my uncle was gay. Not only had he not been a part of our lives because he was gay but he had not been a part of our lives because our personal and familial theology did not make room to even talk about him.

His life was not just dismissed by us, it was invisible to us and yet we were the best he had when that critical time in his life came and he needed somewhere to go. I was thirteen years old. What an impressionable and incredible time in life and I knew watching the death and dying process of my gay uncle — whose sexuality we never openly acknowledged — and whose death we lied about saying he died of liver cancer. I watched his process and determined then that that felt, for me, like injustice. I also recognized then that I also was a gay man. I had never really known what was different about me but something clearly always had been. Over time, I began to understand that there was something about

that intersection of difference and justice — and later I would understand difference, justice, and healing — that would be key to the centrality of my life for the rest of my years.

In 2001, after a lot of life struggle in my own journey I received my own HIV-positive diagnosis. It could have been a crushing moment in my life. But it was not a crushing moment in my life because I had the lessons I had learned from my uncle's experience, and had been in rooms of people like you having an honest dialogue. Together these made space in my heart, spirit, and mind to understand that even after a diagnosis like that, things could, in fact, be different. That actually things today can be different from things that happened before because those miracles are still occurring.

I also know that for those of you who are here with HIV in your bodies, today, that there is a cost for you to be here. That you sit here in this room whether you come out today or any day about your status and you bear an emotional weight and burden that those without the disease do not always understand. I acknowledge you for taking the risk to be here. I honor you for taking the risk to be here and each and every time you do choose to come out I hope you know that there are both the spirits of all who went before us and many of us who are standing on the frontlines of activism who will stand with you in those moments of coming out.

Those of you who are here as allies, I am also aware that it cost you something to be here. This is a piece of the dialogue that we don't talk about enough. It cost something to allow the impact of AIDS to be felt in a meaningful way in our lives.

But the cost of not having the conversation is exponentially greater than the cost of having it.

Can we have agreement on that to start us off?

AMEN! (from audience)

The impact of AIDS fractures relationship with the body, the community, and faith — often requiring radical acts of healing and restoration. Surviving AIDS is, as such, a walk of the spirit. It is an exploration of faith, and a confrontation of our most palpable humanity.

If you are ever confused about the palpable experience of living with and confronting life-defining illnesses, you need only spend some time in a nursing home or a hospice helping someone clean their body, deal with failing body systems and navigating an inability to take care of things that once were taken for granted. This is one of our most palpable experiences of humanity.

It is also one of the moments when we really get it — that if we didn't have a spirit to get us through this there would not be much point in having this thing we walked around in (physical body). We cannot have a spiritual walk without a physical walk and we cannot have a physical walk if we do not include our spirit in the process. So today is both of those things — a walk of the body and a walk of the spirit.

Surviving AIDS is just such a walk and it is serious work. It is significant in its challenge and it demands that we be more than we thought we could be.

So, if we are going to do something serious together it might help if we all did a little homework. I did not want to e-mail it out because I did not know who was coming. And I thought someone would miss the assignment and then you would be embarrassed — tell me your dog ate it. So instead we will take care of it right now. (laughter from audience)

First, I want to note that for the purpose of simplification the acronym AIDS I will use today in place of saying HIV and AIDS. It saves time and I don't have much time with you.

It is relevant to note that it is important at times to distinguish between the two terms. Today we are going to talk in broader brushstrokes about the impact of AIDS which also includes the impact of HIV in our communities, our bodies, and our worlds.

We need to admit a very important and painful truth if we are going to engage this topic. Take a deep breath and listen carefully, please.

AIDS IS NOT OVER.

Can you feel the impact of that statement?

AIDS IS NOT OVER.

We were led to believe a little more than a decade ago that the end of AIDS had arrived when improved medical science and treatments became available in this country and Canada and Europe and in Australia, but...

AIDS IS NOT OVER.

One trip to Africa will clarify this issue for you in a heartbeat.One trip to the impoverished neighborhoods of the United States will clarify this issue. One trip to your local health clinic in any major urban city on World AIDS Day will clarify it for you.

Quite frankly even in those communities where medications are readily available, we know that:

AIDS IS NOT OVER.

Let's try this together — this is the call and response part of the service today.

AIDS IS NOT OVER
(audience repeats)

AIDS IS NOT OVER
(audience repeats)

It is unthinkable that globalization has made the Coca-Cola logo and McDonalds' name brand accessible and recognizable around the world, but there are people who do not know that AIDS even exists — who suddenly find themselves sick and dying and do not even know what is wrong with them — and do not have access to medical care to help them out.

AIDS IS, in fact, NOT OVER.

It cannot be relegated to the history books as something that happened to a generation long gone. It cannot in good conscience be ignored. It cannot be avoided unless we are willing to continue to lose the lives of people around the world, and allow countless others to be permanently altered by a life-defining illness.

AIDS IS NOT OVER.

If you leave here with nothing else to consider as people of faith, I hope you will take that home and have conversation with people around you — and in particular with your peer groups. Then I challenge you to take it out of your peer groups and talk to someone in a different generation. Maybe that is a young person, maybe it is your grandparents, or a cousin or a friend or a coworker. We have to get that message out.

AIDS IS NOT OVER.

Next in our preparation for today, I am going to ask that we attempt to access our spiritual selves to walk together on this path.

Can we agree today to breathe deeply together as an act of prayer, of centering, and of healing? Breathe as an act of community and corporate prayer. Breath is one of those automatic functions of our body that we so often take for granted, but one that those of us with life-defining illnesses cannot take for granted.

Can I breathe with you and ask you to breathe with me?

Let's try it...3 deep, healing, centering, awakening, breaths together.

One... Two... Three

When we enter into a discussion of illness and its impact, it makes sense to remember we do not live in our heads alone. Those of us living with life-defining illnesses, like AIDS, Cancer, Asthma, Diabetes, Fibromyalgia, and many others — the ability to breathe is something that we cannot take for granted. Breath that can be taken away is all the more precious. Breathing can calm the spirit and soothe pain. Breathing in and breathing out can center our spirits and nurture our bodies.

So, today, I ask that we breathe deeply...and at the moments when you feel your emotions reaching that crest and think you don't want to listen anymore, remember to breathe. Something is about to happen to you when you feel a bit uncomfortable.

Finally in our preparation, can we agree to be honest?

I can offer you so much more of what I carry inside me if you are willing to let me be honest and authentic with you. I will need to talk about some hard realities and painful history to guide our walk. And I can receive so much more of what you have to give if you don't wrap it up in pretty wrapping paper — falsehoods — deceptions.

You don't need to look good in this room today. It is okay if you want to cry. It is okay if you want to be angry at the church or me. It is okay to be uncomfortable here. It is also okay to want to celebrate the fact that a seminary is engaging in this conversation, putting its time and money into making something like today happen. It is okay to be happy today.

If we can agree to be in a spiritual space, a space of breath — an act of prayer for us — and an honest place — if we can agree to these things to prepare for the journey, will you join together and say a nice loud AMEN?

(AMEN!)

AIDS challenges the very limits of human compassion and endurance. From its debut as a misunderstood killer of people on the margins of our society to its modern incarnation as a destructive catalyst of change for millions of lives around the world, AIDS has required that people infected and affected by the disease delve deep into our physical, emotional, and spiritual resources for survival.

AIDS has often left us with more questions than answers. Just when it seems we will get ahead of the challenge, a new and harsh reality comes to light.

So there's a tool given to me recently by my physician which I would like to share with you. He is one of the top 100 HIV/AIDS physicians serving the world. He spends 50 percent of his time in patient care and 50 percent working with pharmaceutical companies calling them to ethics and challenges.

I asked him what he thought was the most important thing he had learned. He said the following, "Three words you must learn and be able to use: I don't know."

I DON'T KNOW.

I DON'T KNOW.

If a doctor at the top of his game can say, "I don't know" after almost three decades working to bring an end to AIDS, then how do we find our place in this work when we know there are more questions than answers. AIDS causes us to dig deeply for answers that are simply not always available to us.

What do we need to do to engage AIDS on each of the many levels it impacts our bodies, lives, and communities? How do we resolve the ignorance, misunderstanding, and stigma which continue to so damage the lives of people infected and affected by this disease?

The answers to these questions are not simple, but we can look together at some of the pieces and then spiritually encourage you to look for your own answers.

Admitting that we still don't have a long-term solution to stopping the spread of AIDS nor do we have a cure is a powerful way to access the idea of "I don't know."

Admitting to people now living lives dependent on combination therapies, also known as "drug cocktails," that we cannot predict what other conditions will arise from utilizing these very powerful and often toxic drugs over the course of many years is an act of integrity. It is an act of integrity to say that "I don't know" what will happen to your body after a decade or two decades or three decades.

When my physician told me that the best news he had for me was that he could extend my life by around 25 years — which was a promise my uncle did not receive in 1988 — 25 years because that is the length of time people have been surviving with the support of medications — not even the good medications I have now but the harsh medications from before. "I can guarantee you that we will do everything in our power to give you 25 more years."

I felt grateful for that at the time. Then he said, "The bad news of what I have to tell you is that I don't know what will happen to you over the course of two and a half decades taking these medications. We will have to wait and see."

"I don't know" becomes a very powerful thing to say when it is offered with authenticity and paired with compassion.

Follow it up with the words "I CARE."
"I don't know but I care."
"I don't know AND I care."
"I don't know. I care...about you."

Add to that "I AM WILLING."
"I am willing to be here with you."
"I am willing to hear your concerns."
"I am willing to know your struggle."

"I don't know but I care. And I am willing."

We can all go home now and have a pretty good start with these simple statements and acts.

One of the hardest realities of the early days with AIDS was that we were not in a place where we knew how to say "I don't know" in integrity. It has been a gift of our walk with this disease that we have had to learn those things — how to learn to do them from an honest and open place.

The incredible isolation and stigma that came into the lives of the people who found themselves sick in the beginning had a lot to do with arrogance. It had a lot to with fear and arrogance paired together. It had a lot to do with the fact that we were still willing to subdivide communities up and identify people — you, over there in the third row from now on we will identify you as an agent of contagion and the rest of us will have to be careful about how we deal with you. That didn't feel good did it? For those of us that were in those communities and who continue to live in those communities, every time the label gets attached to the disease we are taken back to the early moments. Many of us were already living in communities that received criticism and shaming messages from members of the dominant culture.

Now...on top of whatever other life challenges we were attempting to overcome, we were sick, too. And the implied message — the not-so-hidden subtext that emerged, was that as human beings we were somehow to be blamed for this illness and its spread in the world — a condition that, in fact, no one could identify an origin for nor clarify how to prevent its transmission. How confusing it must have been in those first few days and how sad that two and a half decades later we are still relatively confused and still have so few answers.

Let's take a look at some points near the beginning...because if we don't review our history, we are doomed to repeat it. Many of us in the room have had a very real experience with this in churches and our communities of origin.

On July 3, 1981, how many of you were above the age of 10? Raise your hand. On that day, the *New York Times* published an article [by Lawrence K. Altman] that would change the lives of one of these groups in the United States, and ultimately around the world, for years to come.

The title read, "Rare Cancer Seen in 41 Homosexuals." It provided a broad and mixed and vague message about a medical condition, which was appearing out of nowhere and seemed to be targeting — they used the word "homosexual" again and again — which seemed to be targeting homosexual men.

Now, in 1972 homosexuality was just being determined to no longer be a mental illness. If my cultural and historical memory had been close to that term being derogatory, this article in the *New York Times*, one of the most legitimate papers in our country, probably would have been hard to see.

The article held very little useful information about how a person became sick with this mysterious cancer or even how to find out if you had it. So, the one overwhelming impression that came from reading the piece was that homosexuals were getting sick with a rare condition. For homophobic and heterosexist readers the labels being attached to the disease indicated that something unhealthy and immoral was creating the circumstance in the homosexuals.

Even before we really knew that sexual transmission was one of the main pathways for the spread of the disease, the very identification of homosexuals as the sick and dying brought up the feelings of sex negativity that existed already in the community and culture.

Author and activist Gayle Rubin in her landmark article, "Thinking Sex: Notes for a Radical Theory of the Politics of Sexuality," keenly addresses these feelings that emerged in that time.

She states, "Most of the discourses on sex [and those ailments which are related to sexual activities], be they religious, psychiatric, popular, or political delimit a very small portion of human sexual capacity as sanctifiable, safe, healthy, mature, legal, or politically correct."

The word "sanctifiable" really got to me. Here she is confronting and critiquing what was happening, and when she used that word, sanctifiable, down in that article she really got to me as a person of faith. Sometimes I get confused about the words moral/ immoral and the more I engage with people of different faith traditions, I realize how lost we get in these words, but sanctifiable gets me right in my Church of Christ roots.

In this model, she notes that there is a sexual hierarchy created by human beings (that's us!) that draws a line between good sex and bad sex. And we take notice of those people — that place between when good sex happens and you don't get sick and bad sex happens and you do.

Rubin continues by saying, "The 'line' distinguishes [the good sex and those having it] from all other erotic behaviors, which are understood to be the work of the devil, dangerous, psychopathological, infantile, or politically reprehensible."

There was a time not long before this in our country, that interracial marriage was being treated in a very similar way, but we don't learn the lessons of history if we don't talk about them.

The reality is that people have sex. In our churches we have to be able to admit that people have sex and talk about the fact that people have sex. All our best efforts have not spoiled that for the human condition. (laughter from audience)

In this model that she is talking about, Rubin challenges us to ask how are we contributing to the drawing of the line between what is good and moral, what is sanctifiable, and what falls in that "other" category.

So, the very morning that edition of the *New York Times* hit newsstands, the lines began to be drawn between the experiences of people with this disease and those people with other diseases, which were "not their fault."

It was implied that it was your fault if you got it by having something on the bad side of the line. It is not your fault if you are one of the other people. Several years later we would get very confused when suddenly there were people who got this disease who did not have "bad sex." They were called "innocent" victims.

Do you know what the phrase "innocent victims" did to those of us on the other side of that line? You can guarantee that we did not go to our doctors, guarantee that we did not seek the help and support and education that we needed, and we did not say what we had because it was bad enough to be on the bad side...but then to be told we were killing children. It was an ugly and dark moment in those times.

August 8, 1982, the *New York Times* published another article, which offered more information. This time they would concretize the perceptions they had only suggested before. I went back and forth and back and forth over the last week about how much of this article to share.

I am going to read the majority of it because there isn't a piece of mainstream literature that came out that year that actually states what was happening more clearly than this. So I want you to listen and I want you to listen in a deeper way. I want you to imagine that, having heard this for the first time, that you are one of the persons it is talking about — that you didn't yet have the disease that was being described but that this cultural and physiological phenomenon was on its way to your life. I want you to imagine that you had one of the physical symptoms being described and didn't even know if you had a doctor who had access to the medical care to help you figure it out.

The title of this article is "A DISEASE'S SPREAD PROVOKES ANXIETY" - By Robin Herman.

It starts like this...

[At this point in his talk, Love quoted extensively from the article which appeared in the 8 August 1982 issue of the *New York Times*. That reading is omitted from this transcript.]

Now those of you who have been around long enough know that there were four groups identified — we often refer to them as the four H's.

Heroin Users, Homosexuals, Haitians and Hemophiliacs.

Those four H's got tossed around and used as a weapon again and again and again during that period of time, with no analysis being done publicly of what this meant to those communities. No analysis about the classism, racism, disease-phobia, homophobia, heterosexism that were implicit in saying the 4 H's again and again — as parts of — say — presidential platforms at the time. But then again, you would have needed a President in the United States at that time who would talk about AIDS and it was Reagan and he wasn't talking.

[Here Love reads another paragraph from the article which describes doctors' theories about the disease's transmission being related to sexual contact and/or blood.]

That was probably some of the most useful information that was provided in the entire article. Then they do something, which was the *New York Times'* attempt to be good and liberal and balanced in the article. They acknowledge that one of the groups working to combat the situation was in fact members of the gay and lesbian community. At the time we mostly said gay community — later we would move into the LGBTQI and allies community, but that is a big progression. Back in those days The National Gay Task Force is noted as coordinating a conference on the disease, and publications for homosexuals, including *The Advocate, Christopher Street* and *New York Native,* had been printing extensive articles about it.

[Quote omitted.]

The article goes on to talk about the anxiety. It goes on to talk about doctors who don't know what to tell people except limiting sexual activity is probably a good idea. It goes on to note that members of the homosexual community appear to be trying to respond to something for which there aren't any answers.

When I read that article, it hits me on a deep emotional level. I can hear all the confusion, pain, and anxiety of the people who suddenly found themselves at the epicenter of a major crisis.

From those pinpoint moments of anxiety and pain, a massive public health and community response began to grow. For those of you interested in truly engaging that portion of the journey, I recommend the book *And the Band Played On* by Randy Shilts. The movie version is very good but misses some very important parts. The book is incredibly comprehensive and worth reading.

While medical experts and community groups like the Gay Men's Health Crisis were scrambling to get accurate data, support the sick and dying, and stop the spread of the disease, other community leaders took this painful moment as an opportunity to lash out at people they disapproved of on moral grounds. These were supposedly people of faith.

Susan Sontag in her brilliant book, *AIDS and Its Metaphors,* offers the following critique of this opportunistic political and religious sort of attack:

"Professional fulminators can't resist the rhetorical opportunity offered by a sexually transmitted disease that is lethal. Thus the fact that AIDS is predominantly a heterosexually transmitted illness in the countries where it first emerged in epidemic form has not prevented such guardians of public morals as Jesse Helms and Norman Podhoretz from depicting it as a visitation specifically aimed at (and deservedly incurred by) Western homosexuals, while another Reagan-era celebrity Pat Buchanan, orates about 'AIDS and Moral Bankruptcy,' and Jerry Falwell offers the generic diagnosis that 'AIDS is God's judgment on a society that does not live by His rules.'"

Sontag was accurate in her criticism of what was happening at that time, but it only scratches the surface of what was happening to faith leaders and those of us in their communities.

As faith leaders, we sometimes fulfill a complicated role in the lives we touch. A harsh and toxic comment from any person in a position of authority may cause undue pain. But when that person of authority can use the power of God as a weapon against a person who is struggling — how much more powerful their argument becomes and how much more powerful the damage!

In turn, I believe our capacity for harm is more than matched by our capacity for healing and hope. If we are not people of a most *UNCOMMON HOPE* then let me ask you this, why are we pursuing lives of faith?

It is important that we look back to those early missteps, cruel intentions and comments if we are going to make a change in the lives of people around the world, today. Because reality is that this is all still happening today.

Musa Dube, an activist and advocate for people living with AIDS in Botswana, reflected recently in the *Global Bible Commentary* (which I hope all of you have on your shelves) in a piece on Mark's Healing Stories, "At the root of all these tough encounters is the social stigma that initially associated HIV and AIDS with sexual immorality, the fear of infection, and the ugly face of death."

Dube's comments in 2000 very much matched what our experience was in the early 80s, describing that people could not leave their homes once they found out they were living with AIDS.

Those insights, those reflections, continue to be true again and again.

So, what is our responsibility to the hidden and invisible people in our communities and families — to the oppressed and the marginalized around us — to our own experiences of marginalization?

What is our responsibility, yours and mine, to the people in our midst and around the world who are impacted by AIDS?

Rabbi Jonathan Sacks in his book *To Heal a Fractured World: The Ethics of Responsibility*

offers the following challenge from the Jewish perspective: "We are here to make a difference, to mend the fractures of the world, a day at a time, an act at a time, for as long as it takes to make it a place of justice and compassion where the lonely are not alone, the poor not without help; where the cry of the vulnerable is heeded and those who are wronged are heard."

Friends, we must ask ourselves and one another if we are taking on the "isms" around us that perpetuate one group or another always wearing a target on our backs and being silenced into oblivion. It wasn't just 1981 and 1982 when we thought it was OK to blame homosexuals for AIDS. It wasn't just 1981 and 1982 when we let people have too little education and information about their bodies to get the health care they need.

AIDS is an opportunity for people of faith, integrity, and compassion to say once and for all...RACISM, CLASSISM, AGEISM, SEXISM, and HETEROSEXISM are not acceptable anymore. The time has come for us to put an end to these things and AIDS is a great opportunity for us — it opens the door for us to say these issues of dividing human beings into categories of isolation and blame MUST STOP.

Bishop John Selders said the following: "When churches start HIV/AIDS ministries as a community outreach service but perpetuate the 'down low,' by not embracing their Same-Gender Loving Brothers in their church pews, we are not serving our people. When white lesbian, gay, bisexual and transgender people are not equally incensed about the growing number of HIV/AIDS cases among poor straight African American women, we are not serving our people. When HIV/AIDS clinics deny treatment to transgender people like Maribelle Reyes in 2007, who died needlessly this year, we are not serving our people. As well as when those of us in the United States refuse to see beyond our own backyard to how this epidemic is destroying entire countries, we are not saving or serving our people."

Those words by Bishop Selders are a really good start on building the *UNCOMMON HOPE* required of us to heal and prevent the further spread of AIDS.

When we get honest and tell the reality of what is happening around the world – telling the truth and saying that we care – and that we are willing. Willing first to talk, next to try and understand from our limited perspectives, and then to take action on what we discover.

That is the place where we begin to build this *UNCOMMON HOPE*. We do not need to live in a world of fractured lives and fractured faith anymore.

People are in need of our stories of hope, our support, and in need of a safe haven.

Labeling, limiting, and subdividing aren't the job we have ahead of us anymore.

How will we stand with the people who are impacted by living with and being affected by HIV and AIDS?

How will we share our stories of hope, strength, and survival in an ongoing age of AIDS?

We can make a good start today by claiming our commitment to *UNCOMMON HOPE*. Each of you is a story that needs to be told. I wish we had a week to tell them in here together.

So, I will ask you to make a commitment to go and tell your story. If you think you do not have an AIDS story, I challenge you to find it. It is not possible to be alive in the world today and not have an AIDS story.

If you think you don't have one, you just aren't asking yourself about it. We all have one.

AIDS has surely been a story with great loss in every chapter, but for every pen stroke of loss there has been a conquest of *UNCOMMON HOPE*.

Will you stand with me, and let me look into your eyes and leave you with this – you my friends, my family, and my community of faith **You are the *UNCOMMON HOPE* of the future. You are the story yet to be told. You are, in fact, the *END OF AIDS.***

article

HIV AND AIDS—CHANGING ALL THE TIME...STILL!

by Joshua L. Love

This article is a blog (www.mccgham.org) entry from August 2008. Love is Director of Metropolitan Community Churches Global HIV/AIDS Ministry.

As I left the 2008 International AIDS Conference in Mexico City last week, I felt in awe once again at the complexity of HIV and AIDS in the lives of people around the world. The impact of this virus has been anything but simple. It complicates the body, mind, and spirit of people living with HIV (PLHIV). I wanted to share a few of the ways our understanding has evolved over time.

On August 3, 2008, the first day of the 2008 International AIDS Conference for which many people around the world had spent days and weeks planning and preparing, a press announcement was released by the United States Centers for Disease Control and Prevention (CDC), which stated the following: "New Technology Reveals Higher Number of New HIV Infections in the United States than Previously Known." This was serious news to those of us working on the frontlines of HIV and AIDS in the United States, and had implications potentially around the world.

I visited the Centers for Disease Control and Prevention website to gather their latest definitions and statistics on HIV and AIDS – I wondered what language the experts are using to explain this multi-layered pandemic. I then went back to a publication, *ALERT*, circulated by Metropolitan Community Churches starting in 1987. Rev. Steve Pieters worked with a team to gather all the information available at the

time and send out updates to the community. I am including for comparison the 2008 CDC definitions and the related 1987 news item from *ALERT*. First you will find the August 3 Press Release from the CDC, then a few excerpts from the CDC website and finally a synopsis written by Rev. Steve Pieters in 1987.

New Technology Reveals Higher Number of New HIV Infections in the United States than Previously Known
Press Release
http://www.cdc.gov/media/pressrel/2008/r080803.htm
The Centers for Disease Control and Prevention (CDC) announced today that an estimated 56,300 HIV infections occurred in the United States in 2006. That estimate differs from the agency's previous estimate of 40,000 because CDC is now using a more precise method for estimating annual HIV incidence, which is the number of individuals who become newly infected with HIV in a given year. The new estimate is published today in a special HIV/AIDS issue of the *Journal of the American Medical Association*, released at the XVII International AIDS Conference in Mexico City.

"These data, which are based on new laboratory technology developed by CDC, provide the clearest picture to date of the U.S. HIV epidemic, and unfortunately we are far from winning the battle against this preventable disease," said CDC Director Dr. Julie Gerberding. "We as a nation have to come together to focus our efforts on expanding the prevention programs we know are effective."

The new estimate is derived from the first national surveillance system of its kind that is based on direct measurement of new HIV infections and builds on a new laboratory test (the BED HIV-1 Capture Enzyme Immunoassay) that can distinguish recent from long-standing HIV infections. CDC's prior annual HIV incidence estimate was based on indirect and less precise methods available at the time.

A separate CDC historical trend analysis published as part of today's study suggests that the number of new infections was likely never as low as the previous estimate of 40,000 and has been roughly stable overall since the late 1990s.

"It's important to note that the new estimate does not represent an actual increase in the number of new infections, but reflects our ability to more precisely measure HIV incidence and secure a better understanding of the epidemic," said Kevin Fenton, M.D., director of CDC's National Center for HIV/AIDS, Viral Hepatitis, STD, and TB Prevention. "This new picture reveals that the HIV epidemic is — and has been — worse than previously known and underscores the challenges in confronting this disease."

Burden Greatest Among Gay and Bisexual Men of All Races and African Americans
CDC's new surveillance system also provides more precise estimates than previously possible of new infections in specific populations. Results confirm that the impact of HIV remains greatest among gay and bisexual men of all races and among African American men and women. In 2006, men who have sex with men

(MSM) accounted for 53 percent of those with new infections (28,700), heterosexuals for 31 percent (16,800), and injection drug users (IDU) for 12 percent (6,600). Infection rates among blacks were 7 times as high as whites (83.7/100,000 people versus 11.5/100,000) and almost 3 times as high as Hispanics (29.3/100,000 people), a group that was also disproportionately affected.

"Too many Americans continue to be affected by this disease," stressed Fenton. "These new findings emphasize the importance of reaching all HIV-infected individuals and those at risk with effective prevention programs."

Separate Trend Analysis Sheds New Light on History of U.S. Epidemic. In addition to the 2006 HIV incidence estimates, CDC conducted a separate, historical analysis that provides new insight into HIV incidence trends over time — overall and for specific populations. Results confirm dramatic declines in the number of new HIV infections from a peak of about 130,000 in the mid-1980s to a low of roughly 50,000 annual infections in the early 1990s. However, findings also indicate that new infections increased in the late 1990s, but have remained roughly stable since that time (with estimates ranging between 55,000 and 58,500 during the three most recent time periods analyzed).

"Prevention can and does work when we apply what we know," said Richard Wolitski, Ph.D., acting director of CDC's Division of HIV/AIDS Prevention. "While the level of HIV incidence is alarming, stability in recent years suggests that prevention efforts are having an impact. In this decade, more people are living with HIV and living longer than ever before due to advances in treatment. Even though this could mean more opportunities for transmission, the number of new infections has not increased overall."

The analysis revealed some other encouraging signs of progress as well as significant challenges among specific groups. Findings indicated reductions in new infections among both injecting drug users and heterosexuals over time. Yet, the findings also indicate that HIV incidence has been steadily increasing among gay and bisexual men since the early 1990s, confirming a trend suggested by other data showing increases in risk behavior, sexually transmitted diseases and HIV diagnoses in this population throughout the past decade. The analysis also found that new infections among blacks are at a higher level than any other racial or ethnic group, though they have been roughly stable, with some fluctuation, since the early 1990s.

"These data confirm the critical need to revitalize prevention efforts for gay and bisexual men of all races and to build upon the growing momentum in the African American and Hispanic communities to confront HIV," said Wolitski. "We must all remember that we are dealing with one of the most insidious infectious diseases in history. Reducing this threat will require action from everyone — individuals at risk, community leaders, government agencies and the private sector."

For more information on HIV prevention, visit *www.cdc.gov/hiv or www.aids.gov*

Basic Information
http://www.cdc.gov/hiv/topics/basic/index.htm#hiv

Brief History
HIV was first identified in the United States in 1981 after a number of gay men started getting sick with a rare type of cancer. It took several years for scientists to develop a test for the virus, to understand how HIV was transmitted between humans, and to determine what people could do to protect themselves.

In 2008, CDC adjusted its estimate of new HIV infections because of new technology developed by the agency. Before this time, CDC estimated there were roughly 40,000 new HIV infections each year in the United States. New results shows there were dramatic declines in the number of new HIV infections from a peak of about 130,000 in the mid 1980s to a low of roughly 50,000 in the early 1990s. Results also show that new infections increased in the late 1990s, followed by a leveling off since 2000 at about 55,000 per year.

AIDS cases began to fall dramatically in 1996, when new drugs became available. Today, more people than ever before are living with HIV/AIDS. CDC estimates that about 1 million people in the United States are living with HIV or AIDS. About one quarter of these people do not know that they are infected: not knowing puts them and others at risk.

Definition HIV stands for human immunodeficiency virus. This is the virus that causes AIDS. HIV is different from most other viruses because it attacks the immune system. The immune system gives our bodies the ability to fight infections. HIV finds and destroys a type of white blood cell (T cells or CD4 cells) that the immune system must have to fight disease.

Definition AIDS stands for acquired immunodeficiency syndrome. AIDS is the final stage of HIV infection. It can take years for a person infected with HIV, even without treatment, to reach this stage. Having AIDS means that the virus has weakened the immune system to the point at which the body has a difficult time fighting infections. When someone has one or more of these infections and a low number of T cells, he or she has AIDS.

CDC Broadens Definition of AIDS
*by Rev. Steve Pieters, Rev. Elder Don Eastman,
and Gary McClelland, M.D.*
*ALERT: News from MCC on Legislation,
Education, Research and Treatment, September 1987*

"It has been recognized ever since the discovery of the Human Immunodeficiency Virus (HIV) as the cause of AIDS and of sensitive, accurate tests to determine its presence that the original case definition of AIDS was far too narrow to include all the manifestations of the disease. As a result, the statistics which are quoted so frequently in tracking the progress of AIDS have not been truly reflective of the full extent of the disease. In response to this awareness, the Centers for Disease Control in Atlanta, Georgia in its August 14, 1987 newsletter presented a new broader definition of AIDS which is expected to increase the counts by more than 15%. ...

"While the primary goal of the CDC in introducing this expanded definition is for its own benefit – to reflect a more accurate picture of how widespread AIDS is – there is, a much more significantly beneficial impact of the definition on the AIDS patient and that is socioeconomic. Up to this point there have been large numbers of people with significant illness, disability, and even death who were never classified as AIDS because of the narrow criteria which previously existed. Because these patients did not fit the AIDS definition they were excluded from many of the benefits which AIDS patients received (i.e disability, SSI, MediCare, benefits from AIDS organization, etc.) With the more realistic definition of AIDS untold thousands will become eligible for these benefits and will no longer be living their lives in the grey zone – that limbo of disability in the absence of diagnosis.

article

HIV AND AIDS IN 2008

by Moderator Rev. Elder Nancy L. Wilson

The body of this article is a reprint of a message from the Moderator of Metropolitan Community Churches to participants at the XVII International AIDS Conference, held 3-8 August 2008 in Mexico City.

HIV and AIDS is a vastly different experience than when I was a young pastor of Metropolitan Community Church of Los Angeles, in the U.S. in 1986.

Today, HIV and AIDS lives and thrives at the intersection of poverty, violence, oppression, sexism, racism and classism as never before. The forces of globalization, for good and for ill, create patterns and opportunities for HIV and AIDS to either flourish or die.

As queer Christians in Metropolitan Community Churches (MCC), we have a legacy that is also our destiny.

HIV and AIDS impacted us savagely in the 1980s and 90s; it also challenged us to be a community of faith and compassion as never before. It molded and shaped us. It ignited a passion for justice within us; it pushed us out of denial and into activism. It taught us to be healers and it healed us in the process.

As people of faith, we are here at this XVII International AIDS Conference in Mexico City, because we cannot *not* be here.

We have much to share and contribute. And we have a lot to learn from the newer communities that are being battered and shaped by HIV and AIDS today. We are citizens of the world, and people of great hope and heart. We are followers of a Christ who was crucified for his love and solidarity with the poor and marginalized.

In our world, religion can be a force for division or for unity-in-action. We live in a pluralistic world and in times that demand religious mutuality and respect from Christianity, whose history too often has been marred by colonialism and intolerance. The friends and members of Metropolitan Community Churches are committed to building ecumenical and interfaith relationships upon which a healing movement of faith can still be built.

We have our courage, strength and experience to offer, willingness to partner and to risk doing what needs to be done to stop HIV and AIDS from killing generations of people in vastly different cultures and contexts.

We know that silence still equals death and that education and access are the keys to empower people with HIV/AIDS and those who care for and about them.

May this XVII International AIDS Conference be a turning point in the struggle to end HIV and AIDS.

With our prayers and best wishes for every success during your gathering this week in Mexico City,

The Reverend Nancy L. Wilson
Moderator
Metropolitan Community Churches

www.MCCChurch.org

Chapter 1 Questions:

1. How has your understanding of the historical impact of HIV and AIDS changed?

2. What of the information covered in this chapter do you feel most inspired to share with others?

3. In what ways has your personal call to HIV and AIDS service been impacted by your learning?

Chapter 1 Notes:

_____

_____

_____

_____

_____

_____

_____

_____

_____

_____

_____

_____

_____

_____

_____

_____

_____

_____

_____

_____

_____

_____

_____

_____

_____

_____

_____

_____

_____

_____

_____

_____

_____

_____

_____

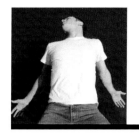

CHAPTER 2

"Our society in general is 'obsexed' – we are obsessed with sex... We can't seem to get enough sex or enough about sex. Those who are not obsessing about how to get it are scheming about how to suppress it."

Christian de la Huerta in *Coming Out Spiritually: The Next Step, 1999*

"For far too long, my view of AIDS, as a black, gay, Christian pastor has been silent. This view has been silent, largely due, I believe, to the view maintained by the uninformed. Why this has caused so much fear within me, I do not know...Fear keeps some of us silent: silent about our sexualities; silent about what we really believe and silent about our health status."

Rev. Leevahn Smith Metropolitan Community Churches

"Stigmatization of persons because of their social status, sexual orientation or addiction to drugs makes them more vulnerable to risks, including the risks of infections. If such persons feel excluded and are afraid of having their identity revealed, they are less likely to seek care and counseling, to have access to health information and to cooperate with AIDS prevention programmes. Thus resistance to all forms of discrimination and advocacy for the rights of people who are vulnerable to HIV are not only ethical demands but also a contribution to effective prevention."

World Council of Churches *Facing AIDS: The Challenge, the Churches' Response, 1997*

Embody: Bodies, Stigma and Wellness in an Ongoing Age of AIDS

Overview of Chapter

All human beings have physical and emotional desires, attractions, and natural longings for companionship. The healthy diversity with which we express these feelings is as complex and rich as the reach of our imaginations. Still for many of us, the ability to talk openly about this vital part of our human experience has been hampered by self-imposed restrictions set up and reinforced by culturally imposed standards and norms. Those of us who have grown up in communities that directly and/or inadvertently communicated messages of shame, stigma, and confusion about our bodies and sexual expressions may experience a literal inability to talk about these issues. When faith-based social norms and HIV prevention messages frame our understanding of human desire in terms of "right and wrong" or "safe and unsafe," we may experience intense emotional pressures to conceal our feelings and life-experiences for fear of rejection.

In this unit, participants are encouraged to *explore their feelings* about their bodies and desires and to *examine the impacts* that HIV and AIDS education and faith-based messages may have had on the development of internal perceptions and community norms related to our physical selves and our sexual identities. HIV prevention messages, particularly those arising from and promoted by faith-based communities, can have results which do not always match their intent: people living with HIV, a medical condition, have sometimes found themselves feeling defined as somehow "less" than people whose bodies do not harbor the virus. In particular, individuals who become infected through sexual contact may hear harsh messages of blame and responsibility from health professionals and religious leaders. The negative feelings and fear of stigmatization resulting from such blaming language can then lead people to avoid HIV testing, to conceal HIV-positive status, to forego support systems and perhaps even to shun medical treatment.

In recent years the tension between abstinence-based prevention models and comprehensive prevention models (which include a range of techniques like condom use, harm reduction, sexual debut delay, etc.), has created a new wave of stigma and concern among people living with HIV and AIDS. In the first session participants examined the external history of HIV and AIDS and its impact on communities. In this session we look more closely at how public efforts to prevent the spread of HIV and AIDS have impacted our relationships to our bodies, our sexuality and self-images. Participants will *explore and examine messages* they may have internalized and adopted from the public discourse, and they will *engage in small- and large-group discussions*, as well as *express their understanding* of body image, sexuality and wellness through an art project.

This unit can lead to a church or public forum on the pairing of sexuality and spirituality. Panelists, perhaps representatives from the church's HIV ministry, can guide the discussion and address how the identification of the body with HIV, AIDS and sexually transmitted infections (STIs) has affected the way we see our bodies and informed our views on the relationship between spirit and sexuality.

AGENDA FOR SESSION

Notes to the Facilitator

Room Set-Up

Full group discussion for the *Uncommon Hope* program works best in a circle if group size permits. If your meeting space will not accommodate such an arrangement, then angled rows from which participants can easily turn to see their peers in other seats will work. It is very important to check on sound and noise levels to ensure that participants will be able to hear presentations as well as each other's comments and feedback. You may wish to break into pairs or small groups for parts of the discussion; if so, plan ahead for any movement of people or furniture. As much as possible, try to anticipate any physical accomodations your participants may need — larger print materials or the services of an ASL or BSL interpreter, for example.

Supplies

This session requires craft supplies including, but not necessarily limited to, construction paper, magazines or similar sources for images/illustrations, rulers, crayons, colored markers, scissors and glue or tape. You may also want to have a large pad of paper or a whiteboard to write on, an easel, a DVD player with speakers for playback, personal inventory sheets, pens or pencils and a notebook for each person which includes paper suitable for journaling.

If you are presenting this session as a stand-alone unit; that is, your participants have not already worked through Chapter 1, you will need to plan for introducing yourself as well as facilitating group introductions. Additionally, you will need to present the *Uncommon Hope* Group Guidelines as part of your introduction to the session. A sample introductory script and a copy of the guidelines begin on page 35 of this book. Be sure to insert the Chapter 2 title, "Embody: Bodies, Stigma and Wellness in an Ongoing Age of AIDS," in place of the Chapter 1 title if you follow the Sample Script.

Session Length

The preferred session length is either 4 hours with a snack or meal break in the middle or two sessions of 2 hours each separated by approximately two weeks. Some participants may want to work on their collages in a non-group setting and/or where they have access to additional art and craft supplies. Regardless of the session length you opt for, do plan on short, hourly breaks. If your session is structured to include a meal, assign small group discussion during that extended break. When people are beginning to know each other, some of the most exciting bonding and sharing can take place in the context of eating together.

Welcome, Introduction of any New Participants and Warm-Up Exercises

Notes to the Facilitator

If you are presenting Chapter 2 as a stand-alone session, this is the point at which you should introduce yourself, facilitate the introduction of participants and read the Group Guidelines. If your participants have already worked through Chapter 1, a quick reminder of the Guidelines, particularly if you have been able to post them in your meeting space, should be sufficient.

Each session of *Uncommon Hope* offers participants the opportunity to explore their own spiritual lives more deeply and to connect more profoundly with others in the group. The process begins at an almost unconscious level when participants first enter the workshop space and becomes overt as individuals share their names a little more formally in the time set for Introductions. To further promote the transition from "outside lives" to the special time of group interaction, you should engage the group in a mindfully preparatory exercise at the beginning of each session. Each community may create its own introductory experiences or you may draw from the activities list provided in the Appendix.

INTRODUCTION TO SESSION 2

Let's talk first about the term Embody and its meanings:

Embody

■ 1 : to give a body to spirit

■ 2 : to make concrete and perceptible

■ 3 : to cause to become a body or part of a body

■ 4 : to represent in human form: PERSONIFY

It is recommended that you have the definitions of Embody posted before you begin this discussion. Alternately, you and the group may "build" the definitions together.

Question for the Large Group

In what ways can we understand HIV and AIDS as an "embodied" experience?

Note to the Facilitator

As the participants respond, write key words and phrases that arise in the discussion on a large sheet of paper or a whiteboard that is visible to the entire group. As much as is practical, continue to display everything you've written throughout the discussion.

Examples can be drawn out by asking some of the following questions to stimulate dialogue:

How does a person get HIV?

Can anyone get HIV?

After a person is HIV+, what changes should he or she make in caring for his/her body?

What messages do you hear when people talk about other people living with HIV and AIDS? Are they positive or negative messages?

What is the best way to foster an environment of safety and support in which people living with HIV can feel comfortable revealing their HIV status?

If you found out you were HIV+ how would you want people to see you? Treat you? Look at your body?

Note to the Facilitator

The following quotes can be used to keep the dialogue flowing in the large group discussion or as prompts for deeper reflection in small group settings. It is suggested that you have these preprinted on posters or slips of paper for participants to read.

Quotes for Reflection on how we experience HIV and AIDS and embodiment

"The genes of the human immunodeficiency virus have engineered a takeover of the factory that is my body. The virus is retooling me to its own use — making copies and reassembling itself. These stray bits of DNA become me, are me, and I am HIV, as much literally in the genetic codes of my cells as in the figurative way that HIV will define me for the rest of my life."

Robin Hardy
The Crisis of Desire, 1999

"When I visit local churches and hear, 'I don't know anyone who is HIV-positive,' I know we are in trouble as a community. I know the people in Metropolitan Community Churches. I live immersed in their stories, so I know it isn't possible for them to not know anyone living with HIV. It tells me that people have stopped feeling safe to 'come out' and tell their stories... that we have returned to the closet."

Joshua L. Love
Director of Metropolitan Community Churches Global HIV/AIDS Ministry
World AIDS Day 2007

"The return to the closet is real. None of the current members of my congregation are public about their HIV-positive status. They're afraid of being stigmatized even in an inclusive faith community. The church has not traditionally been known as a place where you can honestly share your deepest questions and real-life experiences with sex, disease, or drug use."

Rev. Kharma Amos
Metropolitan Community Churches
World AIDS Day 2007

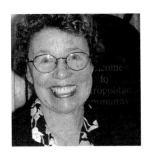 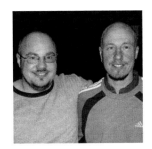 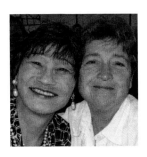 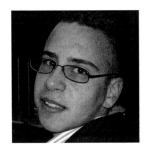

INDIVIDUAL OR SMALL GROUP EXERCISE

Art can be a powerful tool for expressing feelings that may be difficult verbalize or discuss fully. Use the questions below to stimulate creative reflections on the ideas of an "embodied" response and the experience of sexuality and wellness — of seeing HIV and AIDS through new eyes. Then have participants, either individually or in small groups, create collages which represent their perceptions of their bodies: sexually healthy or unhealthy, infected or uninfected, etc. (This might be an opportune moment to remind participants of how practicing both/and thinking can create the possibility for new ideas and perceptions.)

Each participant will need access to art supplies and image sources.

Read aloud or write the questions below where everyone can see them. Ask participants to create images of their bodies as a response to one or more of these questions.

Things to Think About and Questions for Reflection
Do you recognize or identify your body as being vulnerable to HIV infection?

With regard to HIV, what parts of the body seem safe to you?

What parts seem dangerous to you?

Do certain sexual expressions seem safer to you than others?
How did you come to hold these beliefs?

Do certain sexual expressions seem emotionally safer to you?

How do you feel about HIV-positive and HIV-negative people engaging in romantic and/or sexual relationships with each other?

Do you recognize yourself in the media portraits of HIV and AIDS that you have seen or heard?

What do you think the "face of AIDS" looks like today? Is it different now from what it would have been 10 or 15 years ago? If yes, why do you think that's true?

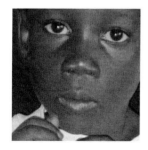 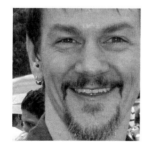 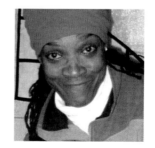 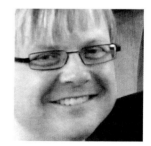

CLOSING MEDITATION/POEM/PRAYER/RITUAL/SONG

Note to the Facilitator

This can be created by the participants or drawn from any resource that is compatible with the faith traditions represented in the group.

Sample

"Here," she said, "in this here place, we flesh; flesh that weeps, laughs, flesh that dances on bare feet in grass. Love it. Love it hard.

excerpt from Beloved *by Toni Morrison, 1987*

For You formed my inward being,
You knit me together in my
mother's womb.
I praise You, for You are to be
reverenced and adored.
Your mysteries fill me with wonder!
More than I know myself do You know me;
my essence was not hidden from You,
When I was being formed in secret,
intricately fashioned from the
elements of the earth.
Your eyes beheld my unformed substance;
in Your records were written
every one of them,
The days that were numbered for me,
when as yet there was none of them.

Psalm 139:13-16 - From Psalms for Praying *by Nan C. Merrill, 2007*

According to Tibetan medicine, a calm and joyful mind will help to balance the four elements — earth, fire, water and air — the building blocks of our body and make the circulation of our energy system function normally. According to this belief, loving-kindness is the best medicine. Along with compassion, sympathetic joy and equanimity, it is one of the four immeasurable attitudes that heal the temporary ills of our life and awaken us.

Tulku Thondup Rinpoche in Shambhala Sun, *March, 2009*

Chapter 2 Questions:

1. Where in your community can individuals go for "safe" HIV testing?

2. What new thing have you learned regarding your feelings about your own body and its health?

3. When you next encounter a person with questions about HIV and AIDS, what will you be most excited to share?

4. In what ways has your personal call to HIV and AIDS service been impacted by your learning?

Chapter 2 Notes:

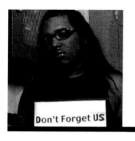

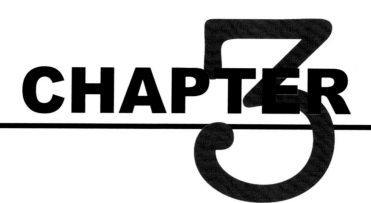

CHAPTER 3

"I know there is strength in the differences between us. I know there is comfort where we overlap."

Ani DiFranco from "Overlap" in *Canon, 2007*

"What a lovely hat belonging is! You walk into the right room, and you pick up this hat and put it on, this hat of belonging, and wonder, what was all that fuss about? The anguish, the loneliness, the lack of connectedness."

Anne Lamott from "Almost 86'ed" in *San Francisco Stories, 1990*

"Sometimes, having lost count a long time ago, I wonder if I know more people who have died than I know ones who are presently alive. Sometimes the line between the world of the living and the alive and the world of the dying and the dead is very blurred for me – as if I, like so many in my community now, live in that strange borderland between the living and the dead, where people are continually crossing over. It is a mysterious and awesome place to live."

Rev. Elder Nancy Wilson Moderator, Metropolitan Community Churches in *Our Tribe, 1995*

Points of Entry: Telling Our Stories

Overview of Chapter

Millions of lives have been lost to AIDS. This painful reality has been changing the course of history — remaking communities, disrupting families, and ensuring that tomorrow will be different from how it was once envisioned. Imagine for a moment that the assassin's bullet had found Rev. Martin Luther King, Jr. before he articulated his dream. Consider a world where Mother Teresa had not lived to see the age of twenty. Hold in your mind's eye the possibility that your own mother or father had not been alive to bring you into the world. Individual lives shape the world — AIDS has taken and continues to take lives, and the world continues to feel the impact.

While there is no way to bring back the myriad possibilities that were lost to AIDS, we can honor the change in our world by telling our stories. We are a different people in the world today because AIDS has ended the lives of men, women, and children who once held the promise of tomorrow. Their life stories — like their deaths — when retold by our witness, have the power to change the future.

The *when* of our entry into an awareness of AIDS and its impact on the world dramatically changes our ability to build context and make meaning. Likewise, our point of view about the reality and weight of AIDS in the world is dependent upon whether or not our personal experience encompasses knowing a person living with HIV and/or AIDS or having known a person who died. To put it bluntly, the experience of a 50-year-old who has lost a loved one to AIDS is categorically different from that of a 20-year-old who has never met an openly HIV-positive person. The first of these individuals has experienced AIDS as a life-altering event, full-force and memorable. The second has perhaps understood that AIDS is one of many serious concerns in the world today like war, recession, homelessness, or terrorism.

The relevance of AIDS is best shared through the direct experience of people living with and affected by the illness. Because of all the people we've lost, storytelling is our best chance to bridge the gap between the past and the future. Those of us who are survivors carry not just our own experiences, but also the life stories of all those we've buried. We hold the possibility of a figurative reincarnation in our willingness to remember and speak. Lives can be saved and futures restored by the simple act of speaking our memories aloud. Where did HIV and AIDS first intersect or merge with your life journey? How has it changed you? What story do you need to tell?

AGENDA FOR SESSION

Notes to the Facilitator

Room Set-Up

Full group discussion for the *Uncommon Hope* program works best in a circle if group size permits. If your meeting space will not accommodate such an arrangement, then angled rows from which participants can easily turn to see their peers in other seats will work. It is very important to check on sound and noise levels to ensure that participants will be able to hear presentations as well as each other's comments and feedback. You may wish to break into pairs or small groups for parts of the discussion; if so, plan ahead for any movement of people or furniture. As much as possible, try to anticipate any physical accomodations your participants may need — larger print materials or the services of an ASL or BSL interpreter, for example.

Readings

In order to derive maximum benefit from this session participants will need to have access to the personal stories at the end of this chapter in advance of the meeting time. It is recommended that they read them all if there is time. If not, then have them select several that "grab" their attention. Each story can be copied from this facilitator's guide; many of them can be downloaded from *www.UncommonHope.org* for email distribution.

Supplies

This session requires copies of the personal stories selected from the resource section at the end of the chapter, pens and/or pencils and a notebook with paper suitable for journaling for each participant. Additionally, you are advised to have plenty of tissues on hand along with several small trash receptacles.

If you are presenting this session as a stand-alone unit; that is, your participants have not already worked through at least one other chapter of *Uncommon Hope*, you will need to plan for introducing yourself as well as facilitating group introductions. Additionally, you will need to present the *Uncommon Hope* Group Guidelines as part of your introduction to the session. A sample introductory script and a copy of the guidelines begin on page 35 of this book. Be sure to insert the Chapter 3 title, "Points of Entry: Telling Our Stories" in place of the Chapter 1 title if you follow the Sample Script.

Session Length

This section of *Uncommon Hope* will require more than one session, thus the total time and number of sessions necessary will vary depending on the size of the group. It is recommended that participants begin to experience speaking their memories aloud in a single session scheduled for about 2 hours. Additional sessions (2 to 4 hours in length) will be needed after participants have had time to work on writing their own stories. Bearing full witness to each person's story may take longer than the exercises in the previous chapters.

For optimal results in the later sessions, it is recommended that you plan for as much as 20 minutes per person for participants to tell their individual stories and experience the empowerment of being respectfully heard. Regardless of the session lengths you opt for, do plan for hourly breaks of 10 to 15 minutes. If a session is structured to include a meal, assign small group discussion during that extended break. When people are beginning to know each other, some of the most exciting bonding and sharing can take place in the context of a eating together.

Welcome, Introduction of any New Participants and Warm-Up Exercises

Notes to the Facilitator

If you are presenting Chapter 3 as a stand-alone session, this is the point at which you should introduce yourself, facilitate the introduction of participants and read the Group Guidelines. If your participants have already worked through Chapter 1, a quick reminder of the Guidelines, particularly if you have been able to post them in your meeting space, should be sufficient.

Each session of *Uncommon Hope* offers participants the opportunity to explore their own spiritual lives more deeply and to connect more profoundly with others in the group. The process begins at an almost unconscious level when participants first enter the workshop space and becomes overt as individuals share their names a little more formally in the time set for Introductions. To further promote the transition from "outside lives" to the special time of group interaction, you should engage the group in a mindfully preparatory exercise at the beginning of each session. Each community may create its own introductory experiences or you may draw from the activities list provided in the Appendix.

INTRODUCTION TO SESSION 3

This unit helps participants to identify their own entry into awareness of HIV and AIDS and to develop a group understanding of their shared cultural experience. It can also be a great tool for preparing people, clergy and laity alike, to offer HIV and AIDS testimonials or to speak before a congregation or other assembly.

All participants are invited to submit written versions of their stories for inclusion on the *www.UncommonHope.org* website of the Metropolitan Community Church Global HIV/AIDS Ministry.

GROUP EXERCISE 1

Tell the group your story. How was your life first impacted by HIV and AIDS? Include as many external details (who, what, when, where, etc.) and internal details (thoughts, feelings, reactions, etc.) as you can recall and feel comfortable sharing.

Note to the Facilitator
If you have 10 or fewer participants, this exercise may be done with everyone in a single group. 15 or more participants should be divided into smaller groups for this activity. If you have between 10 and 15 individuals, you may sub-divide or not depending on your assessment of the likely group dynamics.

Encourage the members to express, in as much detail as possible, the variations of their stories. If participants have difficulty, you may find some of these or similar questions helpful:
- Where did you live at the time?
- How old were you?
- Is this a personal experience or a media story?
- If a media story, did you know an HIV-positive person at the time?
- Do you remember the first experience you had with an AIDS-related death?
- In general, what was the public level of awareness about HIV and AIDS at the time?
- At the time, where might you have looked for more information about HIV and/or AIDS?

INDIVIDUAL & GROUP EXERCISE 2

Before the next meeting, read several of the personal stories included in the resources for this chapter. Reflect on those stories as well as what has been shared among your *Uncommon Hope* group, and then write your own story. Record your first encounter and experiences with HIV and AIDS — the written version of the story you shared aloud — and then extend your story to include details of your journey with HIV and AIDS since that time.

Note to the Facilitator

Determine ahead of time whether your participants will be sharing their written stories within small groups or with the group as a whole. It is a good idea to have some sort of schedule set for when individual participants will be reading/presenting their own stories. Remember also to allow the group(s) some time for reflection and response after each story or set of stories.

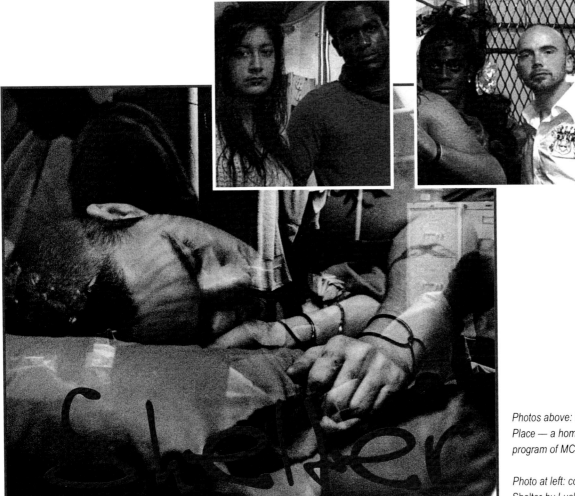

Photos above: from Sylvia's Place — a homeless youth program of MCC New York.

Photo at left: cover of the book Shelter by Lucky S. Michaels.

All photos appear courtesy of Lucky S. Michaels.

CLOSING MEDITATION/POEM/PRAYER/RITUAL/SONG

Note to the Facilitator
This can be created by the participants or drawn from any resource that is compatible with the faith traditions represented in the group.

Sample

> *Thirty-Three Million and Counting: A Psalm for World AIDS Day 2008*
>
> Thirty-three million and counting,
> Each one known to you,
> Each one loved by you, O God.
> As if the population of Canada or Algeria
> All living with HIV.
>
> I thought it would be over now.
> Yet, last year, 2 million died.
> I am stunned into silence by these numbers
> But, silence equals death
> I hear the cry coming back to me across the years.
>
> God, of justice, where is the justice?
> God, of mercy, where is the mercy?
> God, of liberation, where is the liberation?
>
> We cry out to you in anger, in despair,
> In hope of a new day dawning.
> We cry out to you, the names of those we have lost,
> In hope of a new day dawning.
> We cry out to you, for the names added to their number
> Day by day by day.
>
> When did pleasure turn to pain?
> When did freedom turn to fear?
> When did loving turn to hate?
>
> God, of justice, bring us justice.
> God of mercy, bring us mercy.
> God of liberation, bring us liberation.
>
> Thirty-three million and counting.
> Each one known to you.
>
> *Lewis Reay, Edinburgh, Scotland, 2008 (used by permission)*

Therefore prophesy, and say to them, Thus says God: I am going to open your graves, and bring you up from your graves, O my people; and I will bring you back to the land of Israel. And you shall know that I am God, when I open your graves, and bring you up from your graves, O my people. I will put my spirit within you, and you shall live, and I will place you on your own soil; then you shall know that I have spoken and will act," says the Beloved.

Ezekiel 37:12-14
NRSV (adapted)

Photo below "Charlene" :
from Sylvia's Place — a homeless youth
program of MCC New York.

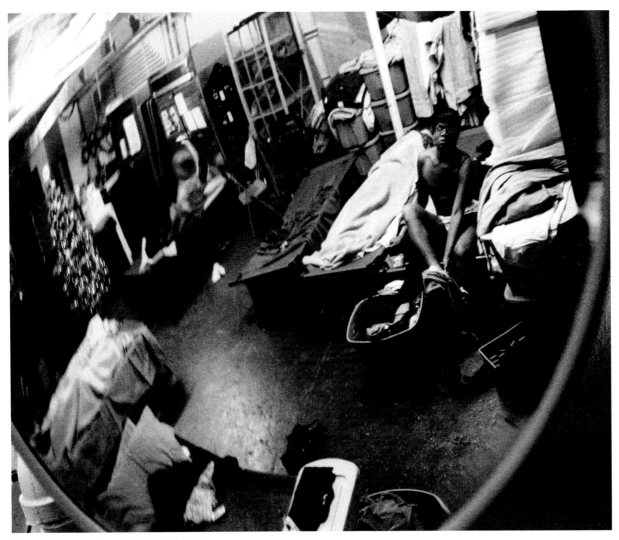

Photo appears courtesy of Lucky S. Michaels.

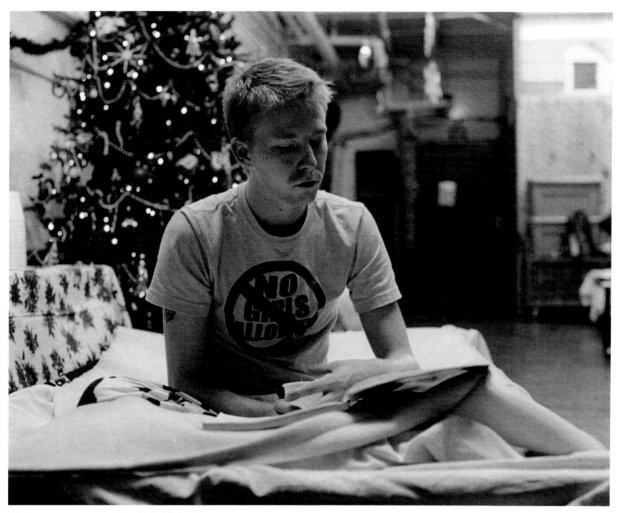

Photo appears courtesy of Lucky S. Michaels.

Note to the Facilitator
In addition to the stories reprinted here, there are useful resource materials listed in the Bibliography and Suggested Readings at the back of this book. The identification and compilation of resources for this unit is an ongoing process. As that body of support materials grows, and in particular expands to reflect a greater diversity of experience and viewpoints, newly available resources will be posted to the Chapter 3 section of the website *www.UncommonHope.org.*

Selections
AIDS at 25
by The Reverend Dr. Troy Perry

As I See AIDS
by Rev. Leevahn Smith

God at the Breaking Point an HIV/AIDS Story
by Rev. David Mundy

Because of Patrick, Another Chance to Get It Right for All of Us: Reflections on HIV/AIDS 2006
by Rev. Dr. Cindi Love

The World, and the Work of the World: Reflections on HIV/AIDS at 25
by Rev. Elder Nori Rost

Reflections on HIV
by Rev. Roland Stringfellow

3 Reflections on HIV and AIDS
by Rev. Elder Nancy Wilson
Excerpted from *Our Tribe*

article

AIDS AT 25

by The Reverend Dr. Troy Perry
Founder and 1st Moderator, Metropolitan Community Churches
This remembrance was published in
INmagazine; AIDS at 25, Volume 9 Issue 8.

www.frontierpublishing.com

Of the thousands upon thousands of memories I have around HIV and AIDS, the most lasting and powerful is my first. It was the early 80s, and the terms "HIV" and "AIDS" did not yet exist.

I received a call early one morning that Dean Sandmire, a young member of our Metropolitan Community Church, had been admitted to Orange County General Hospital. His diagnosis was GRID — Gay-Related Immune Deficiency, a new disease about which little was known.

I made the drive south from Los Angeles and I'll never forget the sight as I stood outside his door. Warning signs were posted everywhere and I remember thinking it looked like a nuclear accident site. Everywhere, signs warned visitors to wear masks, robes, and gloves before entering the room.

I ignored the signs and walked in without any special clothing — but it wasn't because I was brave. I intuitively knew Dean needed to see me as his pastor, and not bundled and hidden and separated from him.

I had taken no more than three steps into his hospital room when Dean broke down. He began sobbing — deep, primal, fearful, uncontrollable sobs. Slowly I moved to his bedside and cradled him in my arms. At least 15 minutes passed before he could speak.

And when he did speak, his first words were, "I'm dying. The doctors give me five months to live."

I continued to hold him in my arms. I looked directly into his eyes and I said, "Dean, you must remember this: Doctors are not prophets. You are living with this; you are not dying with this." Over and over I repeated these words: "You are living with this; you are not dying with this."

When the conversation shifted, I asked if there was anything I could do for him — and he had two requests. He asked that I bring him a Bible, which I readily agreed to do.

But what he told me next made me angry, or more accurately, it was what the Scriptures call "righteous anger" — that is, anger that is directed at injustice.

He said, "The hospital refuses to feed me. The hospital staff is afraid to come into my room and they won't bring me my food; they're leaving my meal tray out in the hall and I'm not able to get it."

I reminded myself that some matters require prayer. And others require action.

So when I left his room, I took the elevator up to the administrative offices and asked to see the hospital administrator. They buzzed me in, and I didn't wait for the usual pleasantries. The words tumbled out of me. "You're the administrator of this hospital, and I have a church member on the first floor who is so ill that he can't get out of bed, and your staff won't even take his meal tray in to him. Now, you probably don't know me, but here's what you should know: If you want publicity for your hospital, I can get it for you. If your staff doesn't immediately begin taking meal trays to my parishioner, I'll have every TV station and newspaper reporter in Southern California down here to cover this story."

Dean's next meal, and every meal thereafter, was delivered directly to his bed.

Here's what else I remember about Dean Sandmire: He didn't live five months. He lived for four years. And he made those years count. And he became the first person with HIV to testify before the U.S. Congress.

Here is something else I carry with me every day: When he did come to the end of his life, in his final hours, as he was surrounded by friends, among the last words he spoke before he slipped into unconsciousness were these, "Be sure to tell Rev. Perry that I lived with it; I didn't die with it."

Like many in our community, my first experience with HIV involved a fight. And regrettably, it's still true. We're still fighting for funding, and for access to medications, and for government attention to a global crisis, and for understanding about HIV.

But I should tell you this: This is a part of Dean's story that I love. After my first visit, every single day members of our MCC congregation went to spend time with him. I was out of town on speaking engagements, and when I returned two weeks later I went to the hospital to visit Dean. And I asked if he had any problems with the hospital staff.

And Dean said, "I've only got one problem, Rev. Perry. Every time they come into my room now, they bring another meal tray. They won't stop feeding me!"

It's the way of memories: One memory leads to another. As I think of Dean's life, another memory comes to mind. It's the memory of 17 years ago, when my partner Philip and I went together for an HIV test and we discovered that Phillip was HIV-positive. HIV has lived with our family, and in our home, all these years.

Dean Sandmire set me on the road to fight for AIDS and he taught me a lesson I still preach everywhere I go: I contend that we all have AIDS. If not in our bodies, we carry it in our hearts.

article

AS I SEE AIDS

by Rev. Leevahn Smith

Everyone seems to have a view about AIDS. I overheard some views just the other day. One view, it seemed to me, expressed a much uninformed, narrow-minded view. Another participant offered an informed, enlightened view of AIDS. Immediately, I felt triumphant, as if I had said it myself. Since I was an observer watching these views unfold, I kept my views to myself.

What is my view of AIDS? Up until now, my view has been silent. Perhaps that is the difference between being an observer and being a participant in life. The observer sits back and watches as life happens for the participants. I offer my view of AIDS now as a participant in life.

For far too long, my view of AIDS, as a black, gay, Christian pastor has been silent. This view has been silent, largely due, I believe, to the view maintained by the uninformed. Why this has caused so much fear within me, I do not know. This same uninformed, narrow-minded view has generated fear with some folks in the black same-gender-loving community and with folks in the African American community as a whole. Fear keeps some of us silent: silent about our sexualities; silent about what we really believe and silent about our health status.

As I see AIDS, from one living more than seventeen years with the virus, I too hold a liberated view of the disease. Liberated in what sense? Participating in safer sex but not sharing my health status is no longer acceptable. Could this be what kept me from taking a stand against the uninformed views of AIDS? By my actions, I was just as uninformed. For that, I wholeheartedly apologize.

My view of AIDS comes from a background rooted in a history of denial, unbelief, mourning, acceptance, support groups and passing. I forgot those other stages when I got to the "passing" stage. In passing, I passed for someone who was not affected by HIV. In my ignorance, I failed to communicate my health status. I stood behind the old facade, as if I was in the current day military, "don't ask, don't tell". I passed right on by the uninformed view, failing to correct the ignorance due to my own. And I passed right on by the enlightened view, telling myself that that view spoke for the rest of us. But I was too afraid to share my view.

No longer can we let these uniformed, narrow-minded views of AIDS keep us in fear. We can no longer be silent about the epidemic of ignorance that dominates the African American community when it comes to the subject of AIDS. I'm reminded of Queen Esther, a Hebrew Testament character who saved her people from being murdered. In her story, no one was permitted to speak to the King without prior permission. Even though she had not been summoned, in order to save her people, she went to see the King. I like how she put it, "And if I perish, I perish." Our community is being annihilated by AIDS and by the ignorance about AIDS. The really sad part that gets me is that the ignorance is worse than the disease. We must do a "Queen Esther" and speak up! Silence does equal death.

Moving past the very early stages of denial, the unbelief, the mourning, and the acceptance and entering into the support groups, I finally found stability and sanity in my life. From the support groups, I discovered that I was not alone. I discovered also that there was strength in numbers. In these support groups, I also discovered that I just existed in life as an observer. In the support groups, I discovered how to be a participant in my own life. I started living. There seems to be a mantra in the support group, "Being HIV-positive is the best thing that has happened to me. I was just existing before, now I've started living." I moved from feeling like a victim to taking charge of my own life.

The face of AIDS has changed over the years. Now I want to share my view of AIDS with others, especially those who are newly affected. This group includes black women and especially black youth who must now take charge of their own lives. This is the lesson that gay white men have passed on to us. You must care enough about yourself to do what is necessary to take charge of your own life: protest, write, and Act-Up! Protesting, writing, and acting-up are actions that we can exhibit in order to take charge of our lives. Otherwise, we will again be accused of sitting back and waiting for someone else to come and rescue us. We are not victims! Historically, we as a people are known for our fortitude. We are a people who simply do not lie down and die over a minute disease on our journey. We are overcomers! We do this first, because we have learned to love ourselves and second, because it is the least we can do for future generations.

My view of AIDS is that it is an opportunity, for those who see it as such, to move beyond the narrow-minded definitions we hold of ourselves and become the very best that we are capable of being. The views of the uninformed may never change. What is most important, however, is how we view ourselves. My view of disease is that it moves us out of our limited existence and opens a way for us to move to that place of being where we were created to be. Of course, this is my view as a minister, as an unashamed HIV-positive black gay man, a father, and one who recognizes the power of love and the power of the Almighty Creator. What's yours?

GOD AT THE BREAKING POINT — AN HIV/AIDS STORY

by Rev. David Mundy

If there's one thing that the AIDS years taught me, it's that death is not the end. I've seen it time and time again, the love that doesn't die. Death is not the end. This is one thing that I have learned from being an MCC chaplain: people don't die all at once — it takes a while, the spirit lingers. The breath goes out, there's nothing left. It's kind of shocking really, how little we leave behind.

One of the things I did as part of my training was attend an autopsy, and I can tell you, the body is nothing really, just a shell; there isn't much there once the spirit goes. I see it all the time in the hospital, there's this moment that comes, when there's nothing left but clay, and you can tell the person's gone.

I saw this with my lover George, who died from AIDS in 1994, my first and only lover at the time. The moment came when it was time to go, it was over, really over, you can sense it when it's finished, and yet his spirit stayed and lingered somewhere just nearby.

A lot of us have felt this with a loved one: in the days and weeks and sometimes months afterward, they still seem to be around. I kept turning my head; kept expecting him to walk into the room. Even now I know he's with me; the love we shared is very much alive. That love will never die. George was a very vibrant person, a person who loved life with a passion, and he had no desire to give it up, as tired and sick and worn out as he was. He came to peace with it, as I have, but it took some time.

I actually think God needs us to remember. God lives in us; that's why I'm in MCC today. This was the place where I met God. And it was in the Eucharist, it was at the table, God's feast where all are welcome, that's where I tasted and felt the living God. And I was hungry for it. I was hungry and thirsty for something I couldn't even name, and this is where I found it. The love that never dies.

We don't exist inside ourselves. Human beings are just not self-sufficient. We need to be seen. We need to be known for who we are, or else we don't exist. Our souls reside in other people. What's the worst punishment that we can inflict one someone else? To make them invisible. To put them in the closet and throw away the key.

Have you seen it in someone else's eyes, as they refuse to acknowledge you in the street, refuse to even see you, because you're old, or strange, or weak, or poor, or your very existence is a threat to their sense of self? It's no accident that solitary confinement is the harshest sentence, a lifetime of loneliness, a living hell, reserved only for the most unredeemable.

That's actually where the good news is: that we will live on, we do live on in every person that we touch. You know how it is when you hear the truth, finally hear the truth about your life, publicly acknowledged. It's liberating, and scary and exhilarating all at once. That's happened to me in MCC as well. I felt it when I went to *Angels in America*; I still feel it every time I see *Longtime Companion*, especially the ending, that scene on the beach at Fire Island, when everyone comes back to life. I always cry. That's resurrection, the resurrection moment. I felt it a couple of years after my lover died, when I said to myself, "I'm going to live. I'm not going to forget him, but I'm going to live. It's what I'm meant to do."

In some ways, our people, those of us who can afford it, we're not in the same sort of danger at the moment. It's kind of like we got a temporary reprieve. Not full restoration, but enough to keep us going, most of us. But I still long for that day, I hope I live to see it, that joyful, joyful day when there truly is a cure for AIDS. Not just a delay, or some treatments to buy some time, but a real and actual cure. Won't that be glorious? When we too can say: "Free at last, free at last, thank God Almighty I'm free at last." I don't know how long it will take, it may not actually be in my lifetime, but I do have faith that the day will come.

Imagine graduating from AIDS, once and for all. I think the feeling that God has forgotten you must be the loneliest feeling in the world, and we've all been there at one time or another. For some of us it was around our sexuality, that feeling of being alone in the world. "Where are you? I need you. I need help." It doesn't feel good to be separated, or outcast, or abandoned. Alone with some new information that rocks your notion of who you are.

I have friends right now who are living on life-sustaining medications, living with HIV or other long-term conditions, and dependent on various medicines to keep them going. Life is precious, for most of us, and most of us want to preserve it and enjoy it as long as we can. But I also see people in the hospital every week who are barely living, barely making it, some of them are pretty close to the end, which brings me to my final question of the heart, the last question of all, which is, when have you had enough? When is it time to call it quits and let go? This is a difficult one, and my answer will not be the same as yours, nor should it be. We struggle with this in the hospital all the time: what are the limits of individual freedom and responsibility? Personally, I hate to see people suffer. Mostly the families hope that nature will take its course; that events will overtake them and they won't be faced with having to make the decision for someone they love. These things are hard; there are no easy answers. Hospitals like things to be neat, and clean. Above all, they like to know what to expect. Life isn't always that cooperative.

BECAUSE OF PATRICK, ANOTHER CHANCE TO GET IT RIGHT FOR ALL OF US: REFLECTIONS ON HIV/AIDS 2006

by Rev. Dr. Cindi Love

Eighteen years have gone by since my brother, Patrick Leo Herndon died in Abilene, Texas of complications arising from AIDS. In the spring of 1987, he called me from his place of work in Dallas and asked me to drive from Abilene to accompany him on a doctor's appointment. We were not particularly close as brother and sister. He was a flaming queen and we often distanced ourselves from one another. So, I found the call unusual. I thought he might need money for a medical procedure and wanted me to help provide support. I asked him what he needed and he said, "Can you just come and we'll talk when you get here?" I said, "Sure."

I drove the next day and met him at the physician's office. I remember feeling irritated that he wore red platform high-heel shoes to the doctor's appointment and too much jewelry. When we went inside the examination room, the doctor thanked me for coming, handed me a brochure entitled "Auto Immune Deficiency Syndrome" and asked me if I had any questions. I had no idea what Auto Immune Deficiency Syndrome was, so I quickly scanned the information. Before I finished reading, the doctor said, "You'll need to make arrangements for Patrick to come home with you."

I said, "Why?" The doctor said "He won't be able to take care of himself soon."

I said, "Why? What is the treatment? Can he not have it here? The hospitals are better in Dallas than in Abilene."

The doctor said, "We are trying to get AZT for him, but it won't help the inevitable progress of the disease. It may make it easier for him to swallow."

I said, "Swallow? What do you mean?" I then turned to my brother and said, "Can you not swallow?"

The doctor said, "He has thrush." (Another word that meant nothing to me except I remembered that infants sometimes had it.)

The doctor said, "He is dying. You have to take him home. I am sorry. I have other patients to see."

I said, "There has to be a treatment. Where can we get it? I'll pay. I don't care what it costs." (At this point I assumed that my brother's insurance was an issue of some kind.)

The doctor said, "There is no treatment. I am sorry." And he left.

My brother was just sitting still in a chair in the examination room. He hadn't said anything at all. The doctor left the room. I said, "Patrick, what is wrong? What does he mean there is no treatment? We can go to Mayo or MD Anderson if we need to."

He said, "It won't do any good. I have a disease that guys like me get. There isn't any cure. Most guys die within a year and I've had it for at least six months. I need your help. My boss is trying to fire me because I missed too much work and if he does, I won't have any disability pay. There is some question whether they will even count what I have as a disability. I can't make my mortgage payment without my pay."

I remember thinking that his mortgage didn't seem like the biggest issue at that moment, but I said, "We'll take care of that. Don't worry."

Then I said, "How did you get this disease? Is it contagious?" (I was thinking about my two children at that moment and my mother who had terminal cancer.)

He said, "It isn't contagious, but they told me that we can't share dishes and you can't be exposed to my blood or any body fluids. I think 'D' gave it to me — that B*&%#! He gave me this and then went back to his wife and kids because his mother said she wouldn't let him come home anymore if he didn't come back to his wife and play the piano at the AME Church."

And then we cried.

Six months later, Patrick died. I did take him home and my mother and dad, sister, my two children and I took care of him. I confess that my parents and my children did a much better job than I did. I wrote the checks and fought his employer (and won!) and avoided my brother as much as possible. Yes, it is true. I avoided him.

Patrick had dementia at the end of his disease process and he was really angry. I caught a lot of that anger because my mom was dying as well

and she couldn't visit him for long periods of time. They were so close and it just broke her heart to see him suffering. One night I went to see him and he jumped out of bed and said I was the Angel of Death. He pulled out all of his IVs and the nurses had to wrestle him back into bed. I felt like I was watching a movie in slow motion. I had no idea what to do and I was scared to touch him.

The nurses caught him as he ran down the hall. After a shot of morphine, he settled down and was resting again. The nurses were cleaning up the room. There was a lot of spilled blood and urine. One of them asked me if I was alright. I had backed up against the wall in the room and was basically frozen in place. I said, "He hates me." She said, "No, he doesn't. He doesn't know what he is saying." I said, "Yes, he really does. I might as well be the Angel of Death because I haven't been an angel of any other kind for him."

You see, after we brought him home, I used Patrick's anger and my mother's heartbreak and my work as excuses for visiting both of them infrequently and turning aside his pleas to get together more. In reality, I was terrified and ashamed and angry and sad. By the time he was nearing the last days of his life, I was pretty frazzled. I was financially supporting my mother (who died six months after Patrick did) as well as my father who had diabetes and was trying to take care of my mother and my brother at home. Three of my business partners were threatening a hostile take-over of the company I founded. And, then there was the issue of my son, Joshua.

Joshua was thirteen years old when he watched the whole story of our family unfold — our fear, Patrick's anger, our shame, Patrick's blame, our love, our grief, and our clumsy and often pathetic attempts to care for Patrick while fearing that we would contract the disease.

Joshua suffered in silence because he knew that he too was gay.

Not long after Patrick and my mother died, Joshua attempted to take his life. I understand his thought process. If I thought my mother, my grandmother and my grandfather and the entire town in which I lived couldn't sort out their issues any better than we did, I would be scared to live. And, he was really close to my mother. Like my brother, he shared her love of art and people and parties and beautiful clothes. He was devastated when she died. And I was distant and working out my life one compartment at a time each day. Not much support for him at all.

Because he was a minor and had tried to take his life, he had to go to local treatment center. The psychiatrist brought me in and asked me if I knew that my son had "gender identification issues." Then he asked me if I had gender identification issues. If a person could die of acute anxiety, I would have died then. Because you see, I am a lesbian and I wasn't out. My gay brother was dead. My gay son tried to kill himself. All I could think of was a ball of twine unrolling and spilling down a set of stairs and I couldn't catch it.

I did manage to get Joshua out of the treatment center where they clearly were not interested in helping him with his depression, but were titillated by the fact that they had a "gay specimen" to study. Maybe even two! And one of them was on the Board of the Chamber of Commerce. (That would be me!) In a way, it helped me that we had an adversary. The fact that the psychiatrist so clearly wanted to capture our ink blots and was willing to entrap my son for as long as our insurance would last infuriated me.

I helped Joshua move to Santa Fe where I owned another business. He lived with one of my employees while he finished his GED. He became the youngest volunteer for National Coming Out Day there and some wonderful lesbians "adopted" him and mentored him and helped him come to terms with who he was. He attended a workshop named "The Experience" about coming out and he invited me to come. The rest is history. I went and came out. My partner, Sue, went and came out. My daughter, Hannah, went and came out.

Then we made a panel for Patrick and we all went to Washington to place it with the AIDS Quilt. The panel carries his name and the span of his life and these words:

Because of you,
Another chance
To get it Right
For all of us.

Patrick's death blew the door wide open on our secrets. I still feel sad that I didn't know how to love him just as he was, but I feel really glad that he helped all of us get real about who we are. Now I can love completely.

I feel sad that there was no treatment for him, but I feel really glad that our family is involved in helping people get treatment today.

Sometimes, I feel sad that my son, Joshua, now has HIV because it is a hassle for him and it may shorten his life, but I am no longer afraid of HIV and I am no longer afraid of the day that death comes for any of us.

I feel really glad that we are no longer as sick as our secrets in our family. I feel really glad that we've "made it through" with one another.

I know now that both body and soul can be witnesses in a way that heals families and makes them stronger and more loving. Patrick lived his life out loud before the rest of us were ready. He was a witness to living with integrity and with love and compassion and I am proud that he was my brother. I am really proud that Joshua is my son and Hannah is my daughter and Sue is my beloved spouse and we're all queer. We have the best time together now. I am happy that Patrick is in a place where I think he can see us. I think he is smiling because all those Queens that used to make me so nervous are now our friends. My mother and he are probably walking hand in hand. Life is good.

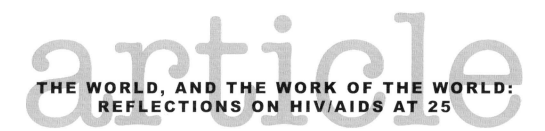

THE WORLD, AND THE WORK OF THE WORLD:
REFLECTIONS ON HIV/AIDS AT 25

by Rev. Elder Nori Rost

A while back, Joshua Love asked me to share some of my thoughts about AIDS as we face the 25th anniversary of its presence in our midst. I had some ideas of what I might say but never enough time to sit down and write them out.

Today, being determined to sit down and actually begin to write, I felt in need of spiritual sustenance so I bought Mary Oliver's book, *The Leaf and the Cloud* [DaCapo Press, 2000]. It's a slim book comprised of a long poem broken into separate stanzas and parts. I had read parts of it before and knew it was one I wanted in my library.

Coming home from Borders Bookstore, I sat on my patio and opened the book and read this quote on the fly leaf:

We have seen that when the earth had to be prepared for the habitation of mortals, a veil, as it were, of intermediate being was spread between them and its darkness, in which were joined, in a subdued measure, the stability and insensibility of the earth, and the passion and perishing of humankind. But the heavens, also, had to be prepared for mortal's habitation.

Between their burning light, their deep vacuity, and mortals, as between the earth's gloom of iron substance, and mortals, a

veil had to be spread of intermediate being; —which should [bring] the unendurable glory to the level of human feebleness, and sign the changeless motion of the heavens with a semblance of human [variation].

Between the earth and mortals arose the leaf. Between the heaven and mortals came the cloud. Their lives being partly as the falling leaf, and partly as the flying vapor.
—John Ruskin
From *Modern Painters*
vol. V, part vii, ch. 1

I thought about this in terms of my own role during these past 25 years. Since I came out when I was 16 years old, in 1978, when I first began hearing the disturbing connections between a strange new disease and gay men, I was instantly impacted. Of course, at that time with no effective treatment, with no test, even, to determine if the virus resided in your blood, the time between diagnosis and death was startlingly fast.

I could recount the names of the ones I loved who died. I could talk about my activism, protesting on the steps of the state capital in Sacramento, California, filling bleach bottles to hand out to IVDUs, lobbying locally, statewide, nationally for better AIDS care, more money to research, because for the love of

God we were dying out there, didn't anyone understand that? I could speak of my outrage at the lack of response to the rising crisis. I could share how I witnessed the birth of AIDS hospices, ACT-UP, Queer Nation and the death of so many fine people, the grief that still destabilizes my center, causing unexpected, often unforeseen earthquakes of pain and memories. I could speak of my role as a lesbian, someone in a largely unaffected group, often referred to as God's chosen, given the low rate of sexual transmission between women.

And I have spoken of these things, have written poems, sermons, journal entries chronicling these events, how they impacted me.

Stop a moment, did you feel that? Just then? Another seismic shift, causing tears to overflow… even now, there is still shifting and settling that occurs in my heart, in my spirit, and I think this will never be truly stable ground, this valley of memories lying squarely on the fault line of AIDS that snakes a jagged line through my life.

And I sense the stability and insensibility of the earth, and the passion and perishing of humankind intertwined, threading through these past 25 years, tendrils reaching into the future still, not just here but globally. So many leaves have fallen from the Tree of Life. So many autumns too early observed. If I close my eyes, I can see them still…these are not the muted shades of brown or yellow, these are the brilliant shade of aspen leaves, who cling to the tree in defiant, burning, fiery glory and, when they surrender to the call of gravity at last, surrender to the need for new life to occur, they spiral down, they dance, it is not defeat but a glorious interpretative dance of life. I remember them at this time of year, when the leaves dress the finely mown lawns in my neighborhood in a ragtag coat of many colors.

Their lives, their love, their insistence on not leaving quietly but in a blaze of glory, grounds me, settles the earth beneath my soul.

And I see them in the clouds, soaring high, shading us from too much light, floating by in huge puffy forms, hinting at the heaven that waits just beyond.

And, here I laugh. Because I realize there is no veil that separates their reality from mine. And, if I've learned anything from these past 25 years, it's the need to be the intermediary between heaven and earth, it's that we are partly falling leaf and partly flying vapors.

So now, I will read Mary Oliver, read her poetry aloud, read, triumphantly, rebelliously, courageously these words with tears still shining in my eyes, and more to come:

> I will sing for the veil that never lifts.
> I will sing for the veil that begins, once in a lifetime, maybe, to lift.
> I will sing for the rent in the veil.
> I will sing for what is in front of the veil, the floating light.
> I will sing for what is behind the veil — light, light, and more light.

This is the world, and this is the work of the world.

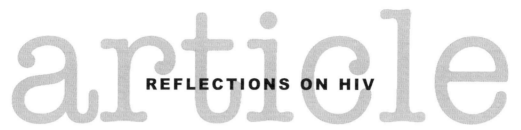

REFLECTIONS ON HIV

by Rev. Roland Stringfellow

How has HIV/ AIDS affected you?
HIV/AIDS has affected me by causing me to be more aware of my sexual practices/partners. It has placed fear in my family members that I may contract HIV and thus they treat me with apprehension. It has led to a loss in friends and mentors who have succumbed to the disease.

How has HIV/AIDS affected the Gay Rights movement?
HIV/AIDS initially devastated the gay rights movement. In the early days of the disease when no one knew how it was contracted or if it was truly a "judgment" of the lifestyle, many people feared one another and even themselves. Some of that fear is still with us. There has been a resurgence in the fight for equality around HIV/AIDS so that people are not left to feel isolated or discriminated against (ACT UP, Stop AIDS Project). Hopefully the gay rights movement will help us all to recognize how we can stop discrimination from within and outside queer communities.

How has HIV/AIDS affected your artistic peer group?
We have lost geniuses like Marlon Riggs, Essex Hemphill, and many others in the Black Gay community.

How has HIV/AIDS affected your ethnic group?
HIV/AIDS is the biggest enemy in the African-American community with African-Americans being one of the largest groups to be infected with the disease. There is a fear and concern among Black women who are infected or fear infection from their husbands who engage in same-sex activities and do not practice safe sex.

How has HIV/AIDS affected your spiritual group?
Many in the Black Church have turned a deaf ear or condemned members in their own congregation who are impacted by HIV/AIDS. I see the Black church as contributing to the lack of information and awareness to African-Americans parishioners.

How has HIV/AIDS affected your age group?
Those in my age group have lost out on having mentors to help guide us in being gay (and Black) in America. Living in the Oakland, California area I have heard of the now closed businesses and debunked social groups due to the devastation of HIV/AIDS. I miss the opportunities that "could have been" if HIV/AIDS was not around.

article

3 REFLECTIONS ON HIV AND AIDS

By Rev. Elder Nancy Wilson
Excerpted from Our Tribe

#1

Gay men and lesbians were the ones who started most of the AIDS agencies in the United States during the first decade of the AIDS epidemic. Those organizations were built and are currently sustained by hundreds of thousands of volunteers and volunteer hours. One of the sociological realities that have made this possible is that proportionately fewer gays and lesbians are encumbered with the demands of child care and raising children. But even those who are have been swept into the tremendous community efforts that have cared for hundreds of thousands of ill and dying friends, lovers, neighbors, and strangers. Armies of lesbian and gay angels, gay and lesbian Mother Teresas, feed, clothe, bathe, nurse, hold, hug, touch, carry, and love the sick and dying men, women and children who have AIDS. It's not that straight people have not also been there, done it – but we've done most of it. And we've also done the praying, the memorials and funerals (sometimes when no one else would do them), and the comforting. We've done this in the face of the virulent, religiously motivated homophobia and AIDS-phobia that communicate to the world, "AIDS is God's gift to the gay community."

The need has become overwhelming and many gay and lesbian persons with any leisure time or disposable income have been pressed into service or extra giving in some way for some period of time. For those of us in UFMCC, AIDS has dominated our local church pastoral care services and our community outreach programs for over a decade.

Everyone who serves selflessly in our culture is deemed an "angel" in the popular mind. The term angel, as in "be an angel," has come simply to mean someone who will serve another not for selfish gain and who does it cheerfully, without any expectation of being paid back. Somehow deeds of kindness and charity are beyond what we think we can reasonably expect of other humans. Somehow, "be a human" doesn't conjure up the same warm, open-hearted, giving image!

In fact, "I'm only human" is the great excuse for letting ourselves and others down. It is the all-encompassing excuse for screwing up. What a definition of humanness!

#2

The concept of the communion of saints in Christian theology is the belief that those who die in Christ commune together eternally before the throne of God and that, from time to time, the church experiences their collective witness and presence (Hebrews 12). We might say that this is the way in which Westerners incorporate the ancient (and, in indigenous cultures, nearly pervasive) practice of venerating (or worshiping or honoring) one's ancestors.

In fact, I remember the story of a young man in Germany who was the lover of the German-born pastor of UFMCC Hamburg. This young man had been a "boat person," a refugee from Vietnam. At age eleven he was rescued by Australians and eventually sent by church people to Germany where he was placed in a foster home. John was gay. A Vietnamese gay man, he was now a German immigrant. His religion of origin was a Vietnamese native religion that was based on ancestor worship. He attended one of his first Christian worship services ever in London at an MCC European conference. There, at an AIDS vigil, he heard people calling out the names of those who had died of AIDS, praying for them and their families and friends, naming and mourning the losses. John, for whom English is a third language, was not sure what was happening. He whispered to his lover, a former Baptist pastor, "Are they calling on their ancestors?" It was a very logical and reasonable assumption! Also, there was truth in that question. Hebrews 11 speaks of our "ancestors in faith" and what it means to remember those who die in faith as part of a heavenly community. Many of those who have died of AIDS are our spiritual ancestors, our particular communion of saints.

One of the things that has happened to lesbians and gay men because of AIDS and because of the virtual epidemic of breast cancer among women in the United States and among lesbians is that we have had to experience the death of dozens or even hundreds or thousands of people we have known personally or have known of, who were often our own ages, more

or less. We are experiencing this selective holocaust while the rest of the world goes on with business as usual (meaning the usual, expected, and also horrific losses — car accidents, other illnesses, etc.). There are times when I have greeted my friends and colleagues at UFMCC meetings and we have spent the first five minutes saying, in small talk, not "How are you?" but a litany of "Did you hear? Did you know that James died, that Ginny is in the hospital, that Al is not expected to live the week?" People whose deaths would have had a big impact on my life ten years ago sometimes — terribly, tragically — become a footnote in my day, as in "By the way, Bob died (yesterday, last week, did I forget to tell you?).

In December 1993 we had a very long staff meeting at MCC Los Angeles. At the end of the meeting, we were making prayer requests. I asked for prayers for our young assistant pastor, Dan Mahoney, who was dying of AIDS, and for a young colleague, a student clergy Doug, who had been in a class I had taught. I mentioned that I was going to visit Doug in the hospital the next morning. My associate pastor, Lori, turned to me, put her hand on my arm, and said quietly, "Doug died this morning." I remember the shock wave — like a little electrical jolt — that went through me. She thought I knew already. I didn't. Now I did. And there was the terrible thought that was partially a relief: one less hospital visit to make — then guilt. I was too late: he had left without my visit. How is his lover Bruce doing? I filed those questions in my mind and went home.

The next day I went to the Veterans Administration Hospital business office with my assistant pastor's lover, Patrick, trying to cut through red tape to get Dan into a hospice. This took nearly three hours. While I was at the hospital, my father died. I flew into my office as usual, and a volunteer said, "Your mother has called twice;

she's holding on line one for you now." My mother never calls me at my office. I knew before I answered the phone.

While I was in New York at my father's funeral, Dan Mahoney died. He had been my assistant pastor and dear friend for many years. At his funeral, I learned of the death of two other people whom I knew and of the critical illness of another. Sometime later that month, I realized that Doug's funeral had been held the same day as my dad's. It seemed finally to have happened to me — what had happened to so many of us: the body count got too high, the pile too deep. I had lost track, I couldn't keep up, I keep meaning to call Doug's lover; I think I left a message on his machine; I'm not sure I ever did. Three months later I managed to go over to him and hug him at the funeral of a mutual friend's father. The circle closed for a moment — but only for a moment.

The lines between life and death blur in this process. The less-than-totally reliable rumor mill sometimes has people dead and buried before they're hospitalized! Or it leaves others behind, pitifully long dead before anyone has time to notice. Sometimes when people get ill they shut out their friends and church family. The hardest days for some of us are finally getting through to someone who tells us, "Santiago died three months ago; didn't you know"

Lloyd was an angel, I'm sure of it. I met him through fellow angel Lew. Lew ended up in a different hospital than he usually went to, and afterward I would come to believe that it was so I could meet Lloyd...I was in the lobby, rushing as usual, dressed in my suit and clergy collar, when Lloyd's sister stopped me. Now when I am in a hurry, you have to be very quick and determined to stop me, and she was. She

grabbed my arm, in fact, and said "What kind of clergy are you? I mean," she amended, "what kind of church are you from?"

Well, I looked at her. It was just possible that she was a lesbian. She had spotted me. So I cut to the chase; "I'm with MCC."

She grinned, "I thought so! My brother is upstairs having surgery right now. He has AIDS, and he's having a hard time. Will you see him?" I said yes, got the details, and went back the next day. (My friend, Lew, by the way, was then transferred to another hospital or went home that day, his angelic mission accomplished.)

Lloyd was a little guy, strawberry blond (just like his lesbian sister — my gaydar had been right), with a sweet Southern Illinois/Kentucky country accent. He poured out his heart about dying, about all his worries (ex-lovers and family members, gay and straight, leaned on him a lot). And his business (a West Hollywood drugstore) was really like a ministry to Lloyd. He loved his customers: they were more like clients or parishioners. He felt too needed, too responsible, to die.

Something happened to me when I met Lloyd. For about two years previously I had been nearly unable to cry at all. I might tear up a little, but I could not cry and certainly could not weep, even by myself. I was shut down, with all the compounded grief and anger. The part that could just spontaneously weep or tear up (which had never ever been easy for me anyway) was totally locked away. As I sat with Lloyd, this gentle, little stranger, I held his hand. He began to sob quietly, and the sight of him (I was identifying with his hyper-responsibility) made me cry. The pleasure of those tears (fogging my glasses, wetting my cheeks) was enormous. My crying did not disturb him: it seemed to help him feel not so alone. Together we cried for so many things, including ourselves.

Every time Lloyd went into the hospital, I would see him. And I would hear a little more about this man's life. After crying with him, I cried every day that week, in my car, at home. It became natural and easy to tear up in my office, at hospices and hospitals, even when I spoke or preached. I felt like I had been healed of a disability. Lloyd had helped me in that moment to reopen to my own tears.

We held his memorial service at the juice bar next door to his drugstore. The place was packed with family, friends, and customers. A big poster-size picture of Lloyd in a happier, healthier time dominated the room. Over and over people testified to Lloyd's kindness and generosity. How much he gave and gave away. How he saved their lives, their dignity. How he was more than a druggist — he was a friend, healer, and a brother.

Lloyd is a part of my own communion of saints. Sometimes, having lost count a long time ago, I wonder if I know more people who have died than I know ones who are presently alive. Sometimes the line between the world of the living and the alive and the world of the dying and the dead is very blurred for me — as if I, like so many in my community now, live in that strange borderland between the living and the dead, where people are continually crossing over. It is a mysterious and awesome place to live. You learn how true it is that death is not a moment but a series of moments, a process. And everyone does it their own way. I have sat by the dead bodies of young dear friends, women and men, held their still-warm, gradually cooling hands. Watched their strained and pain-lined faces relax. Miraculously, tenderly they have seemed to grow younger in that twilight moment of release.

It is a great privilege to accompany them to their border crossing. It is also not what I expected to be doing in the fourth and fifth decades of my life. And I'm so enraged and overwhelmed at times that I want to find someone to blame: I want revenge, I want someone to pay for all this needless suffering, including, I guess, my own. Who pays for all this stolen life and stolen time, including my life and time? And then I think of the arrogance of that thought, that complaint. Who guaranteed or guarantees anyone one minute of life? Where do I get off feeling ripped off — especially when I've had the privilege of loving and serving the dying?

I'm not the only one, I've discovered, who has been profoundly, eternally impacted by the untimely death of dozens, even hundreds of friends, colleagues, and acquaintances. Other friends and colleagues report seeing people in public who they are sure, for an instant or longer, are friends who have long since died. Now and then I will have a powerful sensory memory of someone and then check the date: it's their birthday or the anniversary of their death.

#3
"Send Them"
The days prior to Christmas are always very busy in any church, and that is no less true for those of us at Metropolitan Community Church. Advent is often a frenzied time, as we try to add a dimension of piety, reflection, and centeredness to the cultural holiday bombardment. Since the industrial revolution in the West, and especially in the United States, Christian pastors seem doomed to fight this battle against commercialism, putting Christ back into Christmas, sometimes guilt-tripping our people as they try to walk their own tightropes of overspending, overeating, overdrinking, and other holiday compulsions.

Not only that, but holidays are a time when Americans are most vulnerable to suicide, in overt or more subtle forms. Pastors get more late-night phone calls: there are more strangers calling for help than usual — for emotional, financial or spiritual help. More folks end up in hospitals and emergency rooms. Funerals are twice as traumatic at holiday time.

This is even more true in minority communities. And it is much more stressful in the gay and lesbian community. Alienation from family and traditional support structures (church of origin, for example) is felt much more deeply during holiday times. Some gay and lesbian people are simply not "out" to their families, and they go home having to be very vague about their personal lives. This brings on feelings of guilt and shame and reinforces a sense of isolation. Also, it may mean that lesbians and gays feel compelled to lie about their relational life, friendships, and social, religious, or political activities. ("What did you say was the name of that church you're attending?") Some just avoid contact with their families. Or perhaps Mom and Dad know but ask you, beg you, please don't tell Grandma, it will kill her! Or don't come out to your fundamentalist brother-in-law. "Let's not argue at Christmas!"

Some people who come out to their families are told not to return home for the holidays — or at any time. Other gay and lesbian couples, patiently trying to give their families space and time to "adjust," go their separate ways for the holidays, stealing a minute or two on an upstairs phone to wish their beloved "Merry Christmas," out of earshot for the family's sake.

Increasingly, there are gay and lesbian couples or individuals who finally get to deal with just the usual family and in-law issues during holiday season! What a red-letter day it is for a lesbian when she realizes that her mother has the same kinds of issues with her brothers'

wives or sisters' husbands that she has with her lover! It is such an ironic sign of acceptance — when this lesbian can deal with ordinary family dynamics that are not primarily about homophobia! We need a family "graduation" ceremony at that point. Ordinary, garden-variety in-law conflicts are such a welcome relief to gay and lesbian couples.

For single gays and lesbians, holidays may be a time when they are pressured to date or marry heterosexually. Another good reason to come out!

Holiday times are a special challenge in our church. In addition to the usual Advent services and midmonth church and staff Christmas parties, we hold workshops designed to help people "beat the holiday blues." We go Christmas caroling at gay bars, in hospices, and we try to provide alternative family events, helping people deal with their present status vis-à-vis their families and providing extra support. Some people leave for home for the holidays and let us know they plan to come out to their families. Sometimes that's out of strength of conviction or a need to be honest. Sometimes it occurs in the midst of coming out about HIV or AIDS. In any case, we send people off with promises of prayer, support, and hugs.

We also always offer a Christmas Day Open House. We realized that many times people from MCC would go home after a Christmas Eve service to a long, lonely Christmas Day. Some people need an excuse to leave uncomfortable family scenes ("I'm needed at my church today, Mom!") or a place to hang out, with food and friendly faces.

Ben Rodermond loved food. At special church occasions, he would always bring a treat, something sweet and fattening. His blue eyes twinkled with mischief, his ruddy complexion partially hidden by a Vandyke beard and waxed, old-fashioned handlebar mustache. Soft-spoken and a little shy, he retained his distinct Dutch accent. Ben was a large, tall man who rode a motorcycle, but you instantly sensed he was a gentle, kind person.

Ben loved all kinds of good food, including Indonesian food. He went to Indonesia after World War II. Then he came to the United States, where gradually in the fifties and sixties he began to find other gay people. Ben was there in the earliest days of MCC, feeling a strong, passionate connection to the social Gospel preached by Troy Perry. Even though Ben was not a citizen at the time and was risking more than most people, he stood openly with Troy at the first demonstrations for gay rights in Los Angeles.

Ben also loved food because he knew what it was to be hungry. Ben and his sister Henny and other members of their family had hidden Jews in their home in Holland during the Nazi occupation.

To avoid being conscripted into the Nazi army, Ben went underground for many years as a teenager. Part of the time he hid in a small attic crawl space, while his sister brought him what little food they had, along with news from the BBC. Part of the time he roamed the streets and nearly starved to death there. But he survived. He survived and eventually found friends, gay and lesbian brothers and sisters, and a spiritual home at Metropolitan Community Church of Los Angeles. He had no patience for injustice, for bigotry of any kind. And he had a permanent sweet tooth. Back to my story...

I try to schedule very little during Christmas week, just to leave room for the unexpected and to be able (while choirs are rehearsing, deacons are decorating the church, logistical problems are being resolved!) to be free to reach out beyond our church walls a little to those who are more marginalized, especially in this season.

So that was how I happened to meet Michael on Christmas Eve, 1992.

We had three Christmas Eve services scheduled for that evening, two in English and one in Spanish. The bulletins were done. The church on Washington Boulevard was filled with evergreens. We prayed that it would not be too cold (as it can get in the L.A. desert climate), as our inadequate heater seemed only to taunt us with the hope that it might actually heat up the sanctuary.

My sermons were also done: one for the earlier crowd that included more seniors and people with young children, and one for the more lively "midnight mass" group, on their way to or from Christmas parties or family gatherings. This was one of the occasions in the year when people brought straight parents, children, and family members or gay and lesbian friends who wouldn't be caught dead in church on an ordinary Sunday but for whom it was cool to show up on Christmas Eve.

So I had the entire day free on Christmas Eve, which is what I had planned. There were no last-minute emergencies and only one person in the hospital (which would be my last stop before getting to the church office later that evening).

I decided to stop by three hospices on my way into town. I have always been told by hospice and hospital staff that churches and groups visit patients (especially those without families) all during the weeks up to Christmas but that the visits come to a halt on Christmas Eve and Christmas Day. Most people, including clergy, are simply too busy on those days with their own families and church business. So it felt like my unplanned Christmas Eve and Day visits were more needed and possibly timelier. I set out to visit with a kind of quiet hopefulness, not knowing what would await me.

The first place I went was a hospice I had visited a great many times. At least half a dozen of our members had died of AIDS in this hospice. I knew many of the staff, some of whom were members of UFMCC or who had associations with us over the years. So they didn't look too surprised to see me.

It was a foggy day. The hospice was nestled in a wooded area near a park in downtown L.A. It is a small facility, with a comfortable living room and a devoted staff. This Christmas Eve, it was quiet in a kind of eerie way. When I arrived everything seemed to still. All the holiday hubbub was over before it had begun. There were no family members hanging around as there often are. No music was playing.

I asked the staff if there was anyone who needed a visit from me today. Two staff members looked at each other and communicated non-verbally. Then the nursing coordinator, a man, said, "Well, there's Michael — he's having a hard time." They related to me that they had had a Christmas party the day before. Michael was too upset and maybe too angry and ill to come out of his room. They said that Michael was physically very near death, ready to die, but he seemed anxious and afraid. They knew nothing about his religious issues. But they said, "He just can't let go." They told me he was twenty-five years old and had a sister.

With that little bit of information, I knocked on Michael's door and entered. Even with all the death and dying I had seen, I wasn't quite prepared for this one.

Michael was young. And maybe of average height, but he weighed only about seventy-five pounds. For some reason (unusual in a hospice) he had a nasal-gastric tube and tubes coming out of his mouth and abdomen. He looked a little alarmed when I entered the room. I sat down, told him I was a minister. (I thought my clerical collar might have alarmed him, as in "A clergyperson I don't recognize has come to see me — the end must be near!")

He had a notebook by his head, and he lay facing me on his left side. With his right hand he held a pencil, and I noticed a lot of scrawls on the notebook. Michael was communicating by means of this notebook, since he could not talk with the tubes in his nose and throat. His face was filled with pain and fear. He struggled to position himself so he could write on the notebook. It took quite some time for that to happen. I also realized that he was so weak that he could barely press hard enough to make a recognizable mark on the pad.

I panicked. What the hell was I doing here? I thought to myself. How are we going to communicate? Maybe I'm just frightening him more. I felt guilty for feeling uncomfortable. I wanted to flee from the room. I knew that only Michael, God and I would know the truth if I just left. Whose big idea was it to come here on Christmas Eve, anyway? No normal person would have chosen to be here! Was I trying to be heroic? Brave? A glutton for punishment? And now I was making this kid's suffering worse.

As I thought these thoughts, Michael had finally gotten pencil in hand. "Help," he wrote. Then he pulled on his gastric tube, writhing in pain. Perhaps he thinks the members of the staff here are trying to kill him. Does he have dementia? Or is he just angry, exhausted, a little disoriented with his weakness and the medication? There was no way to know for certain. So I spoke, "Michael, I know you are in terrible pain. No one is trying to kill you, Michael." I touched his head with my hand. "You are dying, and they are trying to help you have less pain and discomfort." At that point, a tear came down his cheek. Michael struggled again to write, with agonizing slowness. He wrote again, "Help me."

I wanted to run. I have never wanted to leave a room so much in my life. Obviously I wasn't getting through, and I was frustrating him. But I touched his head again and said, "Michael, I don't know if I can help you or not. All I can do is pray for you. Do you want me to?" He seemed to nod, I wasn't sure. So I gambled and went for it. I placed both my hands on him and prayed about his fear. I prayed that he could trust God a little more. I prayed for the pain to decrease and cease, for him to be able to relax and trust God, who loved him. As I prayed, I could feel his tears on my hands. Then I felt my own tears.

We opened our eyes. He wanted to write again. This time, the writing came swiftly, mercifully. In a flourish he wrote, "This is a hospice — Christmas Eve. What are you doing here?"

Great question! I had asked it myself about twenty minutes ago. I laughed a little and said, "Well, right now, Michael, I'm crying with you." Then I noticed the Bible underneath his notebook.

"What church?" he wrote.

"Metropolitan Community Church." He showed no sign of recognition. Imagine that — someone in Los Angeles who had never heard of UFMCC! So, as succinctly as I could, I told him the story. I had to assume at this point that it was likely that Michael was gay. I told him I was gay and about Troy Perry and UFMCC. I could see he had never heard of our ministry or about the fact that one could be gay and Christian. His eyes brimmed with tears; he even seemed to smile just a little, in between what looked like electrical jolts of pain. I talked a mile a minute, flooding the room with every reassurance I could manage to speak with confidence. When I took a breath, he wrote, "Angels?" I said yes, I believed in angels and that he had the name of the greatest angel, the archangel Michael. Then he wrote, "Gay angels?"

"Gay angels?" It all came clear. Michael did not want to go anywhere he would not be welcome, including heaven (maybe especially). But if gay angels would accompany him, there was hope! Suddenly I remembered Ben Rodermond from Holland, who had died only three months before in the room next door to Michael's. Ben was an angel, in life and in death. I could see Ben's face suddenly; I could see him coming for Michael, bringing his little gay brother to the throne of grace, holding his hand, healing his fear. "Yes, Michael, there are gay angels: one of them died a few months ago in the next room" I said. Gay angels, what a wonderful thought; the room seemed to be filled with them. "Thank you, God" I kept saying in my heart.

Then Michael wrote again: "Send them."

"Send them." He was ready now, and somehow he thought I had the ability, the authority to send the gay angels for him. So I prayed again for that very thing. Michael seemed calmer. His eyelids rested a little. Gently I touched his face and hands and kissed him goodbye.

That night at the Christmas Eve service, in our very cold sanctuary, we prayed for Michael. I called the hospice the next morning; Michael had died in the wee hours of that Christmas morning, led to his Maker, I'm sure, by Ben and his fellow gay angels.

Chapter 3 Questions:

1. What previously unknown facet or feature of your HIV and AIDS story have you now discovered?

2. Where and how can you share your story in order to make a difference in your community's awareness about HIV and AIDS?

3. In what ways has your personal call to HIV and AIDS service been impacted by your learning?

Chapter 3 Notes:

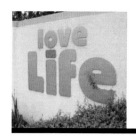

CHAPTER 4

"The only way [to transform perspectives on HIV and AIDS] is to engage with persons who live with HIV. To enter into the life of an HIV-positive person is to walk into a sacred space. It is about sitting and listening, and in so doing, allowing ourselves to be transformed. It is not easy, since one does not know what may happen, and it requires us to come out of our theological boxes. Also, it implies looking more closely at things that usually frighten us, such as sexuality."

Farid Esack   Muslim AIDS Activist, Professor, Theologian and Author

Tikkun Olam Poem

Waiting for the light to come,
In corners of the world,
Some near, some far,
Often no shelter in which to stay...
People who wait, people who pray.

Waiting for the light to come,
Bodies in need of protection,
Villages with freedom lost,
Nations of convicts, militia and strays...
When laws and leaders failed to save the day.

Waiting for the light to come,
Hope born in the heart of a child,
Strength from a mother's love,
Rising from the ashes of each new fray...
Change comes in renewing rays.

Waiting for the light to come,
Awakening a need to help,
Changing focus with open hearts,
Seeing those who are invisible no more...
Connecting to people stepped over before.

Waiting for the light to come,
Until each of us can see,
That the light has been here all along,
Repairing the world and breaking us free...
Changing the Spirit in you and in me.

Joshua L. Love   2007

A Spiritual Walk With HIV and AIDS

Overview of Chapter

The heart of the church is found at the intersection of healing, hope and justice. At the core of the spiritual community are the bedrock values of the love we feel for the marginalized, the compassionate and respectful service we offer those who struggle, and the just attempt to increase our faith by building honest relationships with the diverse people with whom we share this world. Jesus, the central figure of the Christian Bible, modeled and taught that it is our care for one another that should most define our lives together; and that common thread of compassionate concern for all people can be found in nearly all of the world's great faith traditions.

Communities of faith can learn a great deal from the lived experiences and spiritual awakenings born in people living with HIV and AIDS. When people navigate life-defining illnesses each day, their abilities to perceive opportunities for revelation, restoration and a deepening relationship to God are focused through the twin lenses of stress and survival. Spiritual truths rise up, begin to radiate into the community of support around each individual and eventually become accessible to the larger world.

Many churches have struggled with how engagement in the lives of people living with and affected by HIV and AIDS might impact their belief systems. They are confronted with the age-old dilemma of how to extend acceptance and love to "neighbors" whose understanding and application of the spiritual life is different from their own. Perhaps we can help communities of faith to move beyond such concerns by firmly grounding the issues of HIV and AIDS ministry in some of the core teachings of both Christianity and Buddhism:

- "Heal those who are sick...,"
  (Matthew 10:8, *The Inclusive New Testament*, 1994)

- "Aware of the suffering caused by the destruction of life, I vow to cultivate compassion and learn ways to protect the lives of people..."
  (first of The Five Mindfulness Trainings formulated by the Buddhist master Thich Nhat Hanh)

- "So it is with faith. If good deeds don't go with it, faith is dead."
  (James 2:17, *The Inclusive New Testament*, 1994)

Overview of Chapter (continued)

Those who stand in silence while millions become infected and die cannot claim innocence. We face a moral imperative to overcome our own limited points of view; to speak and act in opposition to the destructive forces imperiling so many lives.

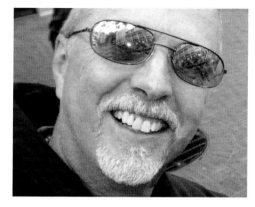

In his 2004 book *Breaking the Conspiracy of Silence*, Rev. Dr. Donald E. Messer wrote, "To date, the efforts of Christian congregations and denominations have been less than minimal. More than twenty years into the global pandemic, most denominations have passed compassionate sounding resolutions but few have become significantly involved in God's mission and ministry of healing." Happily, the past several years have seen the beginnings of a slow shift in the attitudes Rev. Dr. Messer described. People of faith are rallying to find common ground in support of the those who are most impacted by HIV and AIDS and who have precious little in the way of resources to stem the crushing tide of the pandemic.

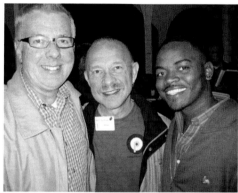

Rev. Dr. Messer said further, "The world may separate us by countries, cultures, races, borders and denominations, but in truth we are all the children of a loving God who cares for every one of us." As people of faith embarked upon a unique spiritual journey, we have an opportunity to transform and heal the world by telling the truth, caring for and about all people and being willing to act where we are needed. No matter how limited our experience or perspective may be, there are ways we can serve to bring an end to HIV and AIDS, to bring an end to the evils of marginalization and to create a world where justice prevails. Where we do this work, we begin to build *UNCOMMON HOPE.*

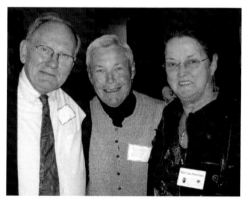

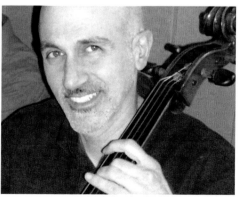

AGENDA FOR SESSION

Notes to the Facilitator

Room Set-Up

Full group discussion for the *Uncommon Hope* program works best in a circle if group size permits. If your meeting space will not accommodate such an arrangement, then angled rows from which participants can easily turn to see their peers in other seats will work. It is very important to check on sound and noise levels to ensure that participants will be able to hear presentations as well as each other's comments and feedback. You may wish to break into pairs or small groups for parts of the discussion; if so, plan ahead for any movement of people or furniture. As much as possible, try to anticipate any physical accomodations your participants may need – larger print materials or the services of an ASL or BSL interpreter, for example.

Reading

In order to derive maximum benefit from this session, participants will need to have access to the Anne Lamott excerpt printed for the Group Reflection Exercise in advance of the meeting time.

Supplies

This session requires copies of the Anne Lamott excerpt, pens and/or pencils and a notebook with paper suitable for journaling for each participant. You may wish to have an easel with a large pad of paper or a whiteboard to write on.

If you are presenting this session as a stand-alone unit; that is, your participants have not already worked through at least one other chapter of *Uncommon Hope*, you will need to plan for introducing yourself as well as facilitating group introductions. Additionally, you will need to present the *Uncommon Hope* Group Guidelines as part of your introduction to the session. A sample introductory script and a copy of the guidelines begin on page 35 of this book. Be sure to insert the Chapter 4 title, "A Spiritual Walk with HIV and AIDS" in place of the Chapter 1 title if you follow the Sample Script.

Session Length

The preferred session length is either 4 hours with a snack or meal break in the middle or two sessions of 2 hours each. Regardless of the session length you opt for, do plan on short, hourly breaks. If your session is structured to include a meal, assign small group discussion during that extended break. When people are beginning to know each other, some of the most exciting bonding and sharing can take place in the context of eating together.

Welcome, Introduction of any New Participants and Warm-Up Exercises

Notes to the Facilitator
If you are presenting Chapter 4 as a stand-alone session, this is the point at which you should introduce yourself, facilitate the introduction of participants and read the Group Guidelines. If your participants have already worked through Chapter 1, a quick reminder of the Guidelines, particularly if you have been able to post them in your meeting space, should be sufficient.

Each session of *Uncommon Hope* offers participants the opportunity to explore their own spiritual lives more deeply and to connect more profoundly with others in the group. The process begins at an almost unconscious level when participants first enter the workshop space and becomes overt as individuals share their names a little more formally in the time set for Introductions. To further promote the transition from "outside lives" to the special time of group interaction, you should engage the group in a mindfully preparatory exercise at the beginning of each session. Each community may create its own introductory experiences or you may draw from the activities list provided in the Appendix.

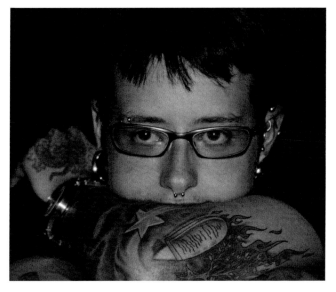
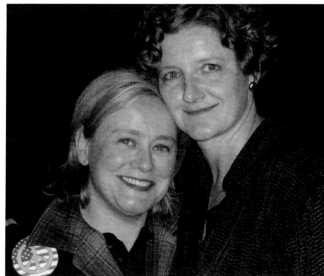

INTRODUCTION TO SESSION 4

In this session, participants take a look at the spiritual elements of HIV and AIDS.

■ What unique dimensions do HIV and AIDS contribute to our prayer lives and our relationships with God, the church and our families?

■ What effect do spiritual and emotional experiences related to HIV and AIDS have on our ability to connect to God and each other?

■ How can our spirituality help us to overcome difficult emotions like despair, anger, depression, and fear?

■ How do we learn to heal the body through spiritual experiences?

■ How can we create safe spaces for an exploration of the spiritual aspects of healing?

■ How does a spiritual support system impact our response to HIV and AIDS, particularly our work for justice, adequate education and medical access for those who are marginalized and most vulnerable to HIV infection?

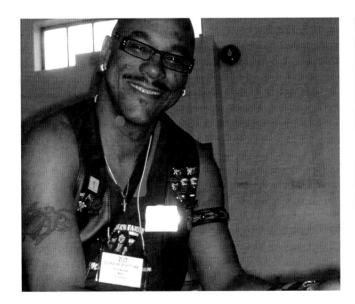 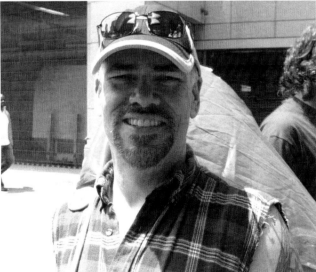

GROUP REFLECTION EXERCISE

The excerpt below is from "Knocking on Heaven's Door" in Part One of Anne Lamott's 1999 book *Traveling Mercies: Some Thoughts on Faith.* After the participants have read the excerpt — if individuals have pre-read as is suggested, you may want to do this re-reading aloud — facilitate reflection on the thoughts and emotions that may have surfaced by posing the questions that appear after the selection.

One of our newer members, a man named Ken Nelson, is dying of AIDS, disintegrating before our very eyes. He came in a year ago with a Jewish woman who comes every week to be with us, although she does not believe in Jesus. Shortly after the man with AIDS started coming, his partner died of the disease. A few weeks later Ken told us that right after Brandon died, Jesus had slid into the hole in his heart that Brandon's loss left, and had been there ever since. Ken has a totally lopsided face, ravaged and emaciated, but when he smiles, he is radiant. He looks like God's crazy nephew Phil. He says that he would gladly pay any price for what he has now, which is Jesus, and us.

There's a woman in the choir named Ranola who is large and beautiful and jovial and black and as devout as can be, who has been a little standoffish toward Ken. She has always looked at him with confusion, when she looks at him at all. Or she looks at him sideways, as if she wouldn't have to quite see him if she didn't look at him head on. She was raised in the south by Baptists who taught her that his way of life — that he — was an abomination. It is hard for her to break through this. I think she and a few other women at church are, on the most visceral level, a little afraid of catching the disease. But Kenny has come to church almost every week for the last year and won almost everyone over. He finally missed a couple of Sundays when he got too weak, and then a month ago he was back, weighing almost no pounds, his face even more lopsided, as if he'd had a stroke. Still, during the prayers of the people, he talked joyously of his life and his decline, of grace and redemption, of how safe and happy he feels these days.

So on this one particular Sunday, for the first hymn, the so-called Morning Hymn, we sang "Jacob's Ladder," which goes, "Every rung goes higher, higher," while ironically Kenny couldn't even stand up. But he sang away sitting down, with the hymnal in his lap. And then when it came time for the second hymn, the Fellowship Hymn, we were to sing "His Eye Is on the Sparrow." The pianist was playing the whole congregation had risen — only Ken remained seated, holding the hymnal in his lap — and we began to sing, "Why should I feel discouraged? Why do the shadows fall?" And Ranola watched Ken rather skeptically for a moment, and then her face began to melt and contort like his, and she went to his side and bent down to lift him up — lifted up this white rag doll, this scarecrow. She held him next to her, draped over and against her like a child while they sang. And it pierced me.

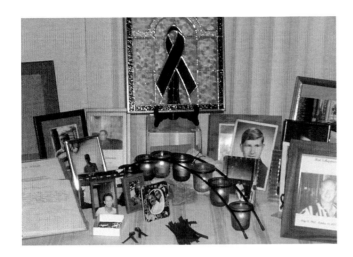 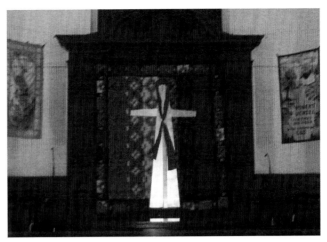

I can't imagine anything but music that could have brought about this alchemy. Maybe it's because music is about as physical as it gets: your essential rhythm is your heartbeat; your essential sound, the breath. We're walking temples of noise, and when you add tender hearts to this mix, it somehow lets us meet in places we couldn't get to any other way.

Reflect

- How do you work to build bridges between people in your faith community?

- Do tensions get spoken aloud? If not, how are they expressed? Are there advantages or disadvantages to these different forms of communication?

- If you are new to the work around HIV and AIDS, what safe places have you found to ask questions about fears and anxieties that may arise when HIV- and AIDS-related topics become a part of the public discourse in your community?

- If you have been engaged in HIV and AIDS for some time, how do you maintain your zeal, find new inspiration and avoid burn-out?

- How often do you utilize prayer, meditation, and singing to bring people together? What other methods or techniques do you think might work to foster solidarity within your community?

SUGGESTED ACTIVITY

Though the experience of a spiritual walk is intensely personal, spirituality may be expressed in a variety of ways — in public, private, individual and / or group settings. An activity that follows naturally from your group's exploration of the spiritual elements of HIV and AIDS is to partner with local organizations or individuals who focus specifically on HIV- and AIDS-related services or who work with and within other vulnerable communities. (Possible partners include, but are not limited to social service providers, medical practitioners, hospital chaplains, local health departments, youth service organizations and various shelter or hospice groups.)

Your partnership might take the form of some ongoing service, say for example providing lunch every 2nd Tuesday or collecting regularly for a food pantry. Your group might provide panelists or support a network of speakers for HIV- and AIDS-focused events or symposia in your area. As your group begins to reach outward, you may well discover needs and develop action plans uniquely suited to your particular setting. Simply establishing points of contact with agencies and entities in the broader community — making known your availability and willingness to serve — can lead to a number of opportunities to share and extend our *Uncommon Hope* in unexpected ways.

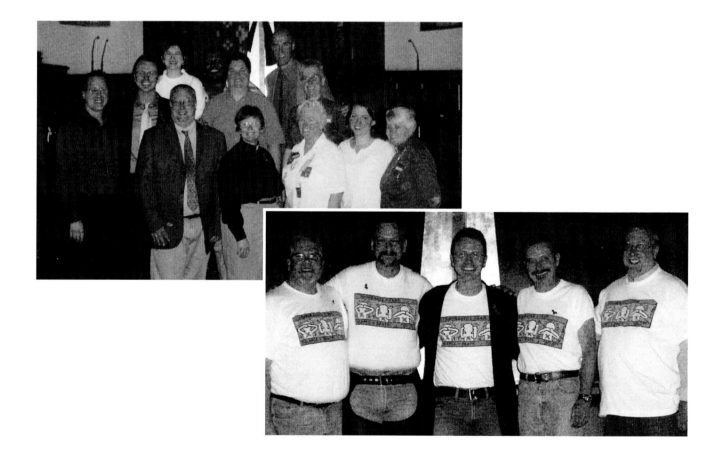

CLOSING MEDITATION/POEM/PRAYER/RITUAL/SONG

Note to the Facilitator
This can be created by the participants or drawn from any resource that is compatible with the faith traditions represented in the group.

Sample Closing Prayer

Holy One —

Bless us with the peace that comes from being still in your presence.
Bless us with an understanding of suffering like the aged who suffer with memory.
Bless us with the compassion of those through whose broken hearts the universe flows.
Bless us with the courage of those who stand alone in the truth of their own lives.
Bless us with redemption equal to the suffering that made it possible.
Bless us with the selflessness of melting snow that becomes invisible with no regret.
Bless us with the determination of rocks and roots and rivers.
Bless us with the faith that believes the sun will rise tomorrow.
Bless us with the uncommon hope that stares at the horizon until it does.

Amen.

Rev. Elder Ken Martin

God gives power to the faint, and strengthens the powerless...God shall
renew their strength, they shall mount up with wings like eagles, they shall
run and not be weary, they shall walk and not faint.

Isaiah 40:29-31

Chapter 4 Questions:

1. What forms of stigmatization and discrimination toward people living with and affected by HIV and AIDS exist in your community?

2. What three concrete steps can you take to make your community safer for and more welcoming of people living with and affected by HIV and AIDS?

3. In what ways has your personal call to HIV and AIDS service been impacted by your learning?

Chapter 4 Notes:

_____

_____

_____

_____

_____

_____

_____

_____

_____

_____

_____

_____

_____

_____

_____

_____

_____

_____

_____

_____

_____

_____

_____

_____

_____

_____

_____

_____

_____

_____

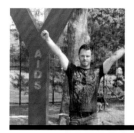

CHAPTER 5

"Sometimes you have to put feet to your prayers."

Rev. Elder Troy D. Perry   Founder and First Moderator of Metropolitan Community Churches

"The New Testament term *kairos*, according to Robert McAfee Brown, refers to a 'time of opportunity demanding a response: God offers us a new set of possibilities and we have to accept or decline'...we affirm an understanding that mission is not something we do if we have a little extra time in the week. It is not just another program of the church or some special outside agency. No, mission is integral..."

Rev. Dr. Donald E. Messer   *Breaking the Conspiracy of Silence: Christian Churches and the Global AIDS Crisis,* 2004

"My walk through the AIDS pandemic has become inseparable from my walk with God. I found the healing power of a loving creator in the harsh reality of HIV and AIDS. I commit myself to serve not just because I am infected and affected by HIV and AIDS but because I am certain that I cannot be a servant of God, a person of faith, if I abandon the millions of people, like me, who will not see another year of life without the support of a massive dedicated coalition of people who care and are willing to take action."

Joshua L. Love   Director, Metropolitan Community Churches Global HIV/AIDS Ministry

"Adversity has the effect of eliciting talents, which in prosperous circumstances would have lain dormant."

Horace   65 BCE - 8 BCE

The *Kairos* Moment: Going Public

Overview of Chapter

Coming to an understanding of our own perspectives, hopes, needs and struggles provides a foundation for right action and best practices which can transform the world. In the previous chapters of this book we have endeavored, through the focused and intentional pairing of spiritual experience and action, to journey into a paradigm that supports first the individual, then the community, and ultimately the world in bringing an end to the AIDS pandemic. Our goal is not small, nor is our work undertaken with a casual attitude. Ending AIDS – like ending human trafficking, environmental degradation, terrorism and warfare – will require significant individual, communal, and global change. The message of *Uncommon Hope* then brings radical clarity to the opportunity Gandhi stated so simply: "Be the change you wish to see in the world."

In the early days of the HIV and AIDS pandemic, the twin specters of fear and death loomed largely unchallenged and no one knew what actions could effectively address the problem. Through fierce attempts to understand the phenomenon, to develop breakthrough medical techniques and to teach strategies for the prevention of new infections, the virulence of HIV and the morbidity rate of AIDS has been somewhat contained, at least in the most privileged parts of the world. A massive infrastructure of coalitions and systems for the support of those persons living with HIV and AIDS has been developed, but even the bravest battles and most stunning successes have not brought an end to HIV and AIDS. There is still no cure.

Now parts of the world less economically and socially privileged, as well as individuals who live in proximity to but have no participation in abundance, provide overwhelming evidence that the work is not complete simply because some lives were saved. In fact, we can affirm with great certainty that until there is a cure, the need continues.

This chapter is about taking action. To borrow some of the language from 12-Step recovery communities: Having had a spiritual awakening, what will you do to make a difference in the lives of others?

■ What inspires you to take action?

■ Where will you commit to serve?

■ What will keep you motivated when difficult circumstances complicate your efforts?

For many of us in communities of faith, there will come a moment when our good intentions are faced with adversity. Perhaps our belief that it is time to form a group of like-minded individuals, rally financial support or raise awareness will be met with the realization that our views are not shared by others. We may find ourselves in groups united by a commitment to action but divided by the ideology of how best to proceed. Some of us may even encounter others who agree philosophically with our positions, but who are unwilling to engage the paradigm shift that will allow thought to grow into reality

Overview of Chapter (continued)

If you take nothing else from this chapter, please accept these words as a gift, from the multitudes of us who have walked this path for the many years of this pandemic: Any action you take is better than passive consent to the loss of one more life to HIV and AIDS. Your missteps and mistakes can open doors to collective action as surely as your successes. Your willingness to act has the potential to transform and heal the world around you. Period.

Recently, a group of HIV and AIDS activists and advocates sat together in a plenary session of an international AIDS conference, listening to a relatively new member of the global coalition dedicated to ending the pandemic. The speaker was emotionally aflame and filled with an obvious, passionate desire to make a difference. The more seasoned workers heard the core message, the subtext of the individual's address, and concern spread among the group that certain aspects of the approach being promoted were perhaps unexamined and/or culturally insensitive — a spiritually motivated individual, poised to leap into action, held the potential to do great good and/or great harm. The group was uneasy and there were rumbles of dissent, but then a wise voice reminded the assembled that each of them once had to take first steps.

Whether you are now facing your first step or are years into your service, you are needed. The *kairos* moment born of the AIDS pandemic is a "time of opportunity demanding a response" in which "God offers us a new set of possibilities and we have to accept or decline." What will you choose?

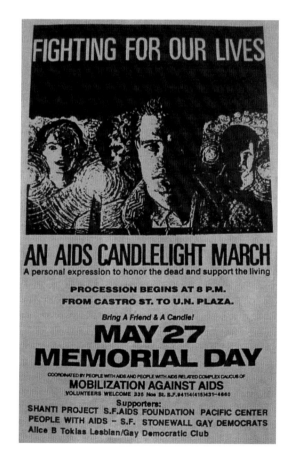

AGENDA FOR SESSION

Notes to the Facilitator

Room Set-Up

Full group discussion for the *Uncommon Hope* program works best in a circle if group size permits. If your meeting space will not accommodate such an arrangement, then angled rows from which participants can easily turn to see their peers in other seats will work. It is very important to check on sound and noise levels to ensure that participants will be able to hear presentations as well as each other's comments and feedback. You may wish to break into pairs or small groups for parts of the discussion; if so, plan ahead for any movement of people or furniture. As much as possible, try to anticipate any physical accomodations your participants may need — larger print materials or the services of an ASL or BSL interpreter, for example.

Readings

In order to facilitate maximum benefit from this session, participants will need to have access to Rev. Farrell's article and the program summaries (that begin on page 142) in advance of the meeting time. It is recommended that they read them all if there is time. The material can be copied from this facilitator's guide or downloaded from *www.UncommonHope.org* for email distribution.

Supplies

This session requires a copy of the readings for each participant. You may also want to have a large pad of paper or a whiteboard, appropriate markers and an easel. Additionally, each participant should have access to journaling supplies.

If you are presenting this session as a stand-alone unit; that is, your participants have not already worked through prior units, you will need to plan for introducing yourself as well as facilitating group introductions. You should present the *Uncommon Hope* Group Guidelines as part of your introduction to the session. A sample introductory script and a copy of the guidelines begin on page 35 of this book. Be sure to insert the Chapter 5 title, "The *Kairos* Moment: Going Public," in place of the Chapter 1 title if you follow the Sample Script.

Session Length

The preferred session length is either 4 hours with a snack or meal break in the middle or two sessions of 2 hours each separated by some time for reflection. Some participants may want to do some "out-of-class" reading or networking. Regardless of the session length you opt for, do plan on short, hourly breaks. If your session is structured to include a meal, assign small group discussion during that extended break. When people are beginning to know each other, some of the most exciting bonding and sharing can take place in the context of eating together.

Welcome, Introduction of any New Participants and Warm-Up Exercises

Notes to the Facilitator

If you are presenting Chapter 5 as a stand-alone session, this is the point at which you should introduce yourself, facilitate the introduction of participants and read the Group Guidelines. If your participants have already worked through Chapter 1, a quick reminder of the Guidelines, particularly if you have been able to post them in your meeting space, should be sufficient.

Each session of *Uncommon Hope* offers participants the opportunity to explore their own spiritual lives more deeply and to connect more profoundly with others in the group. The process begins at an almost unconscious level when participants first enter the workshop space and becomes overt as individuals share their names a little more formally in the time set for Introductions. To further promote the transition from "outside lives" to the special time of group interaction, you should engage the group in a mindfully preparatory exercise at the beginning of each session. Each community may create its own introductory experiences or you may draw from the activities list provided in the Appendix.

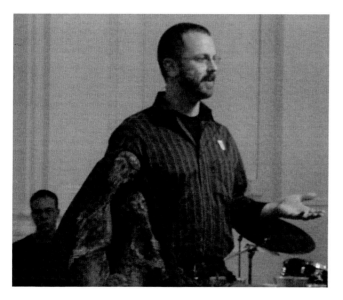
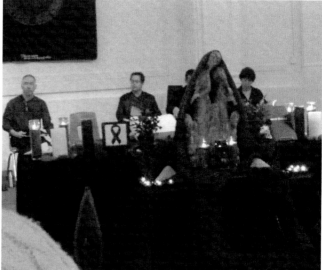

INTRODUCTION TO SESSION 5

In this session, participants visualize and develop service projects and speaking formats for the group to engage in either collectively or individually. A number of opportunities may grow from this session: a powerful HIV and AIDS sermon/worship/testimonial series (with support from the local leaders of faith-based organizations,) AIDS Walk projects, news or editorial series in local media that reawaken community dialogue and response to HIV and AIDS, to list but a few.

GROUP EXERCISE

Have the participants share the article "AIDS — Yesterday and Today: Breaking the Stained Glass" in small group settings. As they complete their reading, ask them to reflect on and discuss their responses to these questions:

1. What stimulated Rev. Farrell's decision to "go public?"
2. What steps did he take to create a public forum?
3. What were the specific outcomes of his actions?
4. How might this type of vigil be constructed in your community?
5. What other kinds of actions would be appropriate to your community?
6. Who would you enlist as partners in the creation of a strong coalition?

(The questions are reprinted at the end of the article)

After participants have discussed the reading in small groups, reconvene the large group and facilitate a comparison and further discussion of the small groups' responses to the last three questions.

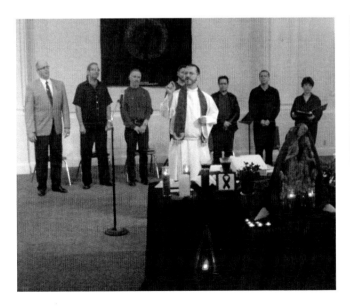
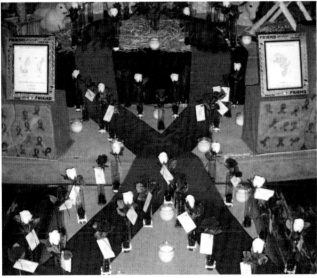

AIDS – Yesterday and Today: Breaking the Stained Glass
by Rev. David Farrell, Pastor Emeritus MCC San Diego, California (USA)

It was wonderful to be an MCC Pastor in 1980, leading a young and vibrant congregation in sunny San Diego, California. I grew up in this fairly conservative, mostly Republican, city by the sea. It had been a small town, but by 1980 it had become (almost without any of us noticing) a vast military/industrial complex, and the 8th largest city in the country. Our healthy, young (average age 25-45 and predominantly gay male) congregation had just completed a successful capital campaign and moved triumphantly into a new church home which was too large for them, when AIDS slipped into San Diego silently as a shadow on a sunny day.

This invisible predator moved swiftly among us...unseen, unnamed, unnoticed... smooth...like a warm knife moves through butter. It left in its wake a narrow corridor of disease and death at the heart of San Diego's gay male community. We would learn to name it AIDS and to know it well as disease and death invaded our church and the community we served.

Death was so new to us. As the founding generation of MCC, we had no real experience of death in our midst at all. There was no elder generation; no normal cycle of life and death. And only the men got sick and died. The example of women in our community rising heroically to minister to us is the proudest story of my generation. For many gay men, the strength and unselfish courage of women during the early years of AIDS dealt a death-blow to any lingering vestiges of male superiority. They were church-goers (or not), they were lesbians (or not); they were our friends, mothers, sisters, mentors, nurses, drivers, shoppers, housekeepers, nurses, cooks and caretakers...they were magnificent, and they were there for us! and I'll never forget it.

We didn't know the cause of AIDS then. There weren't any effective treatments, and it almost always ended the same way. A sudden onslaught of little-known or half-forgotten cancers and other terrifying illnesses would attack a weakened immune system and MCC had another suffering patient (and another funeral) on the way. There weren't really any gay-affirming churches then and it seemed as though everyone in town was coming to MCC for services.

An odd thing happened in all of this. In the beginning, many gay people had been indifferent (if not openly hostile) to MCC and its ministry. The disgraceful ways in which so many churches had shunned us and shamed us and cast us out over the years had crippled many of us spiritually and emotionally, and left us with "a chip on our shoulder" for organized religion. We came by it honestly. I felt it too. But that didn't mean we stopped believing in God, or a higher power, or a life beyond this one.

So, when I visited AIDS patients in the hospital or at-home, they were glad to see me, but as death drew near, their thoughts turned to the churches of their childhood. The young men really wanted a priest, minister, or rabbi from their own religious tradition. Most of them wanted a church burial. They wanted their lovers to be in charge of the arrangements. They wanted their relationships honored. They wanted their friendships and affiliations respected. And, they wanted the cause of their death acknowledged. Our churches had previously denied us all of the above, but things were different now, weren't they? We were dying. Foolishly, perhaps naively, I hoped so. How sad and disappointed I was to learn that, even in the face of suffering and death, young gay men were still being denied the comforts of faith.

In San Diego, MCC stepped into the breach. Never before had our congregation been so challenged. For the first five years, with the help of God, a united community, and a struggling group of home-grown, bootstrapped charities, we did it all...and we were glad to do it. Indeed, I believe God had raised us and strengthened our church for just "such a time as this." MCC was truly the spiritual center of our community.

We were called to perform the "corporal works of mercy"...to feed the hungry; give drink to the thirsty; clothe the naked; harbor the harborless; visit the sick; ransom the captive; and bury the dead. All of us, clergy, boards, deacons, and congregation were ministering with both hands to all comers. Together, we searched for ways to acknowledge the diversity of lifestyles in our community because we had to. We learned a lot about illness and death and relationships because the learning was thrust upon us. We opened our minds and hearts to other faith traditions because we had no choice. And, along the way, we mastered the practices of family counseling and intervention, revolutionized the ritual of grieving, and raised Funeral and Memorial Services to an art form.

I don't mean to say that nobody else was willing to help. I think many other clergy or churches wanted to, and some did. I thank God for them. And there were also clergy from a variety of faith traditions who wanted to help, but were either afraid to, or just didn't know how. Others just kept wishing it would all go away. Some of the more bigoted preachers were at their very worst, taking cheap shots about AIDS being God's punishment for being gay and wallowing in their own sanctimony until their own clergy, their inner circles, and some of their children started dying from it.

By 1985, I was exhausted, overwhelmed and surrounded by fear, death and denial. It seemed few people were talking and nobody was listening. I knew I had to find a way to break through the stained-glass windows of denial that were insulating so many local churches and clergy from facing the reality of this crisis. These were their people too!

In January 1985, I held a press conference to announce that MCC San Diego would be hosting a 50-hour AIDS Vigil of Prayer, beginning on a Friday evening and continuing uninterrupted for 50 hours. The Sanctuary would be open day and night with staff and volunteers in constant prayer. There would be a series of musical presentations and five ecumenical worship services. Our entire property would be devoted to AIDS awareness and education. Every AIDS organization would staff a booth with information about their needs and services. Doctors and nurses would offer the latest AIDS medical information, and legal experts would educate GLBT people about legal remedies available to them. Volunteers and offerings would be raised for the various local AIDS charities. People with AIDS would share their experiences. Every religious leader and every congregation in the city would receive written invitations and schedules and would be personally invited to attend and pray with us at some time during the 50 hours. We wanted to offer an event that would give everybody an opportunity to participate, and give everybody a way to attend.

The weekend came, and male and female clergy from a kaleidoscope of religious traditions showed up in a bewildering assortment of vestments to participate in the various worship services. Prayers were offered; blessings were bestowed; resentments were spoken; confessions were made; apologies were offered and accepted; forgiveness was given...and all the while a steady stream of people crowded our seminars and display booths, and moved in and out of our Sanctuary; praying, listening to music, engaging in quiet contemplation, or writing a message to lost loved ones on the massive AIDS banners placed on the walls for that purpose. Lessons were learned, grief was shared and many people were strengthened and comforted...and for a while there, it was like we know it's supposed to be when the people of God gather together: "Fulfill you my joy, that you be likeminded, having the same love, being of one accord, of one mind." (Philippians 2:1-2)

It was a perfect storm...or the planets were aligned, or maybe it was simply God's will, because it proved to be the right event, in the right place, with the right focus, at the right time, and it worked like a Swiss watch! The church community, the GLBT community, and the larger community responded enthusiastically to the whole idea. Everybody did their part. An outpouring of volunteers, a torrent of free publicity (in both gay and mainstream media), and an overwhelming response from other clergy and churches, all came together in a blessed harmony that stunned us all!

Media coverage before, during, and after the vigil, was massive and uniformly positive. One rabid fundamentalist congregation staged a loud and vulgar protest out in front of church on Sunday morning and received a scorching TV editorial for their efforts. We took a lot of stills and video during the weekend, and got footage of the media coverage from all our local TV stations, and permission to use it in the video we were making of the vigil weekend.

When we shared our video with MCC Fellowship officers, I was asked if our congregation would implement this program fellowship-wide. We were honored to do so. In 1986, MCC San Diego led the fellowship in the very first International AIDS Vigil of Prayer. We created a comprehensive "how-to" kit, with a copy of our video, tee shirts, polo shirts, postcards, even envelope seals with a distinctive Vigil logo. We sent the Vigil Kit to every church in MCC, and I made presentations at several MCC District Conferences.

We didn't know how successful it might be, so imagine our surprise and joy when MCCs around the world embraced the idea wholeheartedly. All of our congregations did it on the same weekend. That meant that prayer, AIDS education and AIDS awareness programs never stopped all around the world for 50 hours on that weekend. As in San Diego, other churches and organizations cooperated and participated in unheard of numbers. When MCCs sent in their final reports and the results were tabulated, we found that over five thousand (5,000+) churches worldwide had participated in the 50 hour International Vigil.

Many say that Rev. Troy Perry and Metropolitan Community Churches have altered the course of religious history. It's true, I think. MCC does change things…it changes minds, melts hearts, and alters the course of people's lives. MCC changed me in dramatic ways, giving me back my faith, my sobriety and health, and my vocation to ministry. That's why we were there when the first waves of the AIDS pandemic hit our communities; it's why we'll still be here when HIV/AIDS is gone.

Who ever dreamed that a Prayer Vigil could be voted "Event of the Year" by a local GLBT community? Well, that's exactly what happened in San Diego, California in 1985. At General Conference in 1987, the MCC Fellowship honored our congregation with an award for the most effective fellowship program in MCC history. And we have taken enormous pleasure and satisfaction in seeing the weekend Vigil of Prayer evolve into the international "World AIDS Day." We didn't know any of this when we started out. We were just taking the next step…just trying to be authentic…just trying to be faithful. That's all we're called to do.

Things to Think About & Questions

   1. *What stimulated Rev. Farrell's decision to "go public?"*
   2. *What steps did he take to create a public forum?*
   3. *What were the specific outcomes of his actions?*
   4. *How might this type of vigil be constructed in your community?*
   5. *What other kinds of actions would be appropriate to your community?*
   6. *Who would you enlist as partners in the creation of a strong coalition?*

SUGGESTED ACTIVITY

Discuss, develop and plan for a specific action in your community.

To accomplish this activity, participants will need to gather and process information about HIV and AIDS programming. It is suggested that they begin this process by reading the five summaries provided below. In addition, participants may want to contact service providers in your community (individuals and agencies, both current and past providers) to determine exactly what needs exist locally and how those needs are or are not being addressed. If other church or faith-based ministries are already operating in your vicinity, contacts with them may prove valuable as well.

These are intended to serve not as models for what your participants might create, but simply as examples of the variety of opportunities available.

The Ezekiel Project

The Ezekiel Project, a ministry of MCC of Greater St. Louis in St. Louis, Missouri (USA), was initiated in the summer of 2006 as an outreach to HIV-positive individuals, their caregivers and allies. The church provides both budgetary support and a staff liaison, but the project is run completely by volunteers. The ministry serves as a social support group and represents the local church in the larger community. Each of The Ezekiel Project's monthly meetings offers a spiritual element as well as an opportunity for social connections.

The group is involved in a number of varied activities:

- sponsoring an annual, no-cost-to-participants, 2-day retreat addressing both spiritual and life needs;
- coordinating MCC of Greater St. Louis' participation in the annual "Dining Out for Life" event where local eateries contribute a percentage of their income to local AIDS service organizations;
- supporting local AIDS service organizations by advertising and participating in their events;
- sponsoring the annual community candlelight vigil in May to honor the memory of those lost to HIV and AIDS;
- participating in World AIDS Day events;
- participating in and providing support as needed for local memorial services;
- maintaining a journal and scrapbook, housed in the church, of people who have been lost to HIV and AIDS.

Another important component of the ministry is the pastoral care that is provided through The Ezekiel Project. People in the ministry provide help and assistance to people in crisis via the church's 24-hour crisis phone line. They also act through informal mechanisms in the church and community to offer support to persons living with and affected by HIV and AIDS.

Additionally, The Ezekiel Project ministry has allowed people to become more open about being HIV-positive. The ministry's leaders feel strongly that coming out fosters healthy relationships, and The Ezekiel Project has been very effective at modeling this often scary practice. Perhaps the most positive thing that has come out of the ministry is the opportunity for HIV-positive people to serve: serve each other, serve the church, and serve the local community.

Information courtesy of Danny Gladden, MCC of Greater St. Louis

The Fellowship Health and Wholeness Ministry

> *The Fellowship is a coalition of churches and ministries from across the USA each affiliate of which has a vision to minister to individuals who live on the margins of society. This group of daring and visionary ministers and ministries is led by Bishop Yvette Flunder, Founding Pastor of City of Refuge United Church of Christ in San Francisco, California.*

The Fellowship Health and Wholeness Ministry was initiated in December 2005 as a means of equipping The Fellowship and its member churches to address adequately the health matters that individuals living on the margins of society are faced with on a day-to-day basis. HIV/AIDS education was the primary focus of the ministry during the first two years because many individuals who are directly and indirectly connected to this conference are African American, same-gender loving men and members of the ever-growing transgender community – groups which, nationwide, have a high rate of HIV prevalence.

The Health and Wholeness Ministry has coordinated several educational sessions on the issue of HIV prevention and care during the conference's Leadership Retreats as well as during General Convocation. These sessions have focused particularly on the rising rate of infection among African American women, African American same-gender loving men and minority youth. Topics addressed included:

- How HIV affects the human body
- Epidemiological data regarding the prevalence of HIV in high risk populations
- Effective methods for building an HIV ministry within the church

Individuals selected to lead and present at various sessions included:

- Representatives from pharmaceutical companies that focus on HIV/AIDS treatment
- A Centers for Disease Control staff member
- Individuals living with HIV/AIDS
- HIV/AIDS ministry leaders
- Staff members of AIDS service organizations from across the nation

In June of 2008 the Health and Wholeness Ministry collaborated with the Dallas County Health Department and Dallas-area community business organizations to provide free, confidential

HIV testing to individuals attending the General Convocation in Dallas, Texas. These efforts were doubly successful in that many people were tested and a number of Fellowship pastors reported they were moved to return to their home churches with a new zeal to begin the work of educating their congregants and the communities in which they serve.

During the 2008 General Convocation, The Health and Wholeness Ministry hosted a luncheon geared toward equipping spiritual leaders to provide effective guidance to new parishioners living with HIV as well as to those who come to them for guidance around the reality of a new HIV diagnosis. Also during the event in Dallas, Health and Wholeness team members worked with the Fellowship's Youth Ministry to provide "HIV 101," a training session designed for teenagers.

The ministry's next step will be to launch a quarterly e-newsletter featuring articles and information about many of the diseases that plague members of marginalized community, including but not limited to HIV/AIDS.

> *Information courtesy of Rev. W. Jeffrey Campbell,*
> *The Fellowship Minister of Health and Wholeness*
> *Bishop Yvette Flunder, Presiding Bishop*

Ribbons of Hope

Ribbons of Hope is a ministry of Vision of Hope MCC in Mountville/ Lancaster, Pennsylvania (USA). The program was organized in January of 2006 and grew, in part, out of dissatisfaction with the fact that the only HIV support group then available in the area had become no more than a forum for public complaint. Though the group is a ministry of the local church, it is funded primarily through grant money and currently receives about $1000 every six months from each of two different drug companies.

Ribbons of Hope meets weekly in rented space (Vision of Hope MCC is not conveniently located for the majority of attendees.) to share a meal, distribute essential items and enjoy social connection. Invited guests often attend to speak on topics of particular interest to the group — a recent guest spoke on prayer — and the group provides pastoral care to members in need. The church's Associate Pastor meets weekly with the group's leaders and attends the meetings once a month to provide support.

In addition to hosting their regular meetings, Ribbons of Hope provides social support to attendees and helps direct people to resources available through other local agencies and organizations. When services are unavailable, group members "fill the gap" as they are able, providing food and even housing in their own homes for persons in need. The group advertises through the church, with local physicians, in the local gay magazine and with other HIV organizations in town.

One of Ribbons of Hope's long-term goals is to see HIV/AIDS housing become available in the city of Lancaster.

> *Information courtesy of Chris Jackson, founder and co-leader, Ribbons of Hope*

No Day But Today

No Day But Today, which takes its name from a song in the musical *RENT*, is a ministry of Wichita Falls MCC, in Wichita Falls, Texas (USA). The program was initiated in 2006 when two of the church's members approached the pastor with their desire for a place where people could discuss issues associated with or related to HIV.

Initially, the group met twice monthly and used the Empowerment Program (an earlier version of *Uncommon Hope*) developed by MCC's Global HIV/AIDS Ministry Director, Joshua Love. No Day But Today currently meets once a month and meetings always begin with a Positive Note: each attendee shares a word or phrase that he or she finds uplifting. A period of discussion and planning follows, during which the group considers both past and future events, and the meetings typically conclude with a time for sharing and/or questions.

Although the group came into being primarily to provide support to people living with and affected by HIV and AIDS, No Day But Today has grown into a second purpose: community outreach. Outreach activities to date have included:

- a forum at the local university entitled, "AIDS? In Wichita Falls?"
- sponsorship of a local HIV/AIDS Walk/Run
- participation in events hosted or sponsored by local AIDS service organizations

The group meets at Wichita Falls MCC and welcomes any interested participants.

Information courtesy of John Forsythe, co-founder, No Day But Today

Bethlehem-Judah Ministries, Inc
an Affiliate of The Fellowship

The HIV & AIDS Ministry at Bethlehem-Judah Ministries, located in Dover, Delaware (USA) began its outreach near the end of 2006. The present focus of the ministry is membership recruitment and HIV/AIDS awareness and prevention.

Due to the fact that most of the ministry members had little to no knowledge regarding actual outreach or HIV/AIDS education, we began our work together by bringing in an Outreach Specialist from a local non-profit organization in Dover to provide some basic training for the ministry members. The specialist conducted several seminars offering information and instruction on several topics:

- the types of and effects of drugs bought and sold on the streets,
- drug users and dealers,
- HIV/AIDS education,
- prostitution,
- demographics of areas hard hit by HIV/AID,
- safety and protection when doing street outreach

The seminars were advertised to other community churches and a representative of John Wesley AME attended the training. Workshop participants received certificates of completion.

The team's next task was to prepare kits suitable for handing out during outreach ventures. The kits were primarily informational — brochures, lists and fact sheets for local housing, help lines, HIV testing sites, detoxification sites and counseling services — but they also contained male and female condoms and a brochure from Bethlehem-Judah Ministries.

Finally, the ministry hit the streets of Dover, Delaware. Outreach ventures were conducted in local housing projects and other areas that have a high rate of drug use and prostitution. While distributing the kits, ministry members also provided community residents with safer sex tips.

As a result of this work, many lives have been impacted in a positive way. The success of these grassroots efforts has opened a door for the church to work with AIDS Delaware and Kent/Sussex Counseling Services.

Information courtesy of Wilford L. Oney, Jr., Pastor, Bethlehem-Judah Ministries, Inc

CLOSING MEDITATION/POEM/PRAYER/RITUAL/SONG

Note to the Facilitator

This can be created by the participants or drawn from any resource that is compatible with the faith traditions represented in the group.

Closing Meditation

The Invitation

It doesn't interest me what you do for a living.
I want to know what you ache for
and if you dare to dream of meeting your heart's longing.

It doesn't interest me how old you are.
I want to know if you will risk looking like a fool
for love
for your dream
for the adventure of being alive.

It doesn't interest me what planets are squaring your moon...
I want to know if you have touched the centre of your own sorrow
if you have been opened by life's betrayals
or have become shriveled and closed
from fear of further pain.

I want to know if you can sit with pain
mine or your own
without moving to hide it
or fade it
or fix it.

I want to know if you can be with joy
mine or your own
if you can dance with wildness
and let the ecstasy fill you to the tips of your fingers and toes
without cautioning us
to be careful
to be realistic
to remember the limitations of being human.

It doesn't interest me if the story you are telling me
is true.
I want to know if you can
disappoint another
to be true to yourself.
If you can bear the accusation of betrayal
and not betray your own soul.
If you can be faithless
and therefore trustworthy.

I want to know if you can see Beauty
even when it is not pretty
every day.
And if you can source your own life
from its presence.

I want to know if you can live with failure
yours and mine
and still stand at the edge of the lake
and shout to the silver of the full moon,
"Yes."

It doesn't interest me
to know where you live or how much money you have.
I want to know if you can get up
after the night of grief and despair
weary and bruised to the bone
and do what needs to be done
to feed the children.

It doesn't interest me who you know
or how you came to be here.
I want to know if you will stand
in the centre of the fire
with me
and not shrink back.

It doesn't interest me where or what or with whom
you have studied.
I want to know what sustains you
from the inside
when all else falls away.

I want to know if you can be alone
with yourself
and if you truly like the company you keep
in the empty moments.

Oriah from her book The Invitation, *© 1999. Published by HarperONE,*
San Frnacisco. All rights reserved. Printed with permission of the author.

www.oriah.org

Do not be conformed to this world, but be transformed by the renewing of your
minds, so that you may discern what is the will of God — what is good and acceptable
and perfect. For by the grace given to me I say to everyone among you not to think
of yourself more highly than you ought to think, but to think with sober judgment,
each according to the measure of faith that God has assigned. For as in one body
we have many members, and not all the members have the same function, so we, who
are many, are one body in Christ, and individually we are members of one another.

Romans 12: 2-5

Chapter 5 Questions:

1. What new or re-established commitments are you willing to undertake to alter the impact of HIV and AIDS in the world?

2. What will you do to sustain your inspiration; how will you maintain your motivation when difficult circumstances complicate your efforts?

3. In what ways has your personal call to HIV and AIDS service been impacted by your learning?

Chapter 5 Notes:

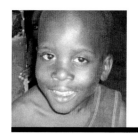

CHAPTER 6

"When it comes to global health, there is no 'them'... only 'us'."

Global Health Council

"We are all sick because of AIDS – and we are all tested by this crisis. It is a test not only of our willingness to respond, but of our ability to look past the artificial divisions and debates that have often shaped that response. When you go to places like Africa and you see this problem up close, you realize that it's not a question of either treatment or prevention – or even what kind of prevention – it is all of the above. It is not an issue of either science or values – it is both. Yes, there must be more money spent on this disease. But there must also be a change in hearts and minds; in cultures and attitudes. Neither philanthropist nor scientist; neither government nor church, can solve this problem on their own – AIDS must be an all-hands-on-deck effort."

Barack Obama   Illinois Senator speaking on World AIDS Day 2006

"The global HIV/AIDS epidemic is an unprecedented crisis that requires an unprecedented response. In particular it requires solidarity – between the healthy and the sick, between rich and poor, and above all, between richer and poorer nations."

Kofi Annan   Seventh Secretary-General of the United Nations

One Body: Gaining a Global Perspective

Overview of Chapter

The work of our sisters and brothers in Zimbabwe to serve children living with and affected by HIV and AIDS is a living expression of faith.

> Joshua L. Love
> *Director,*
> *Metropolitan Community Churches*
> *Global HIV/AIDS Ministry*

The Metropolitan Community Churches Global HIV/AIDS Ministry's commitment to explore new relationships and missions in the global AIDS pandemic took a sizeable leap in the summer of 2005. The denomination's General Conference, a global convocation of member and partner faith communities, met in Calgary, Alberta (Canada) and there — in worship, in conference gatherings, and on the streets of Calgary — stood in solidarity and compassion with people living with and affected by HIV and AIDS around the world.

At that conference the MCCGHAM gratefully accepted the combined invitation of the Yvette A. Flunder Foundation, Refuge Ministries, and The Fellowship to partner in support of an orphanage in rural Zimbabwe. With faith communities in 25 countries spanning the globe, MCC had long had opportunities to offer short-term support to HIV and AIDS efforts around the world, but this new endeavor promoted a new direction for service through an intention to create long-term sustainability.

Rev. Elder Jim Mitulski and Joshua L. Love, now Director of the MCC Global HIV/AIDS Ministry, reminded our fellowship of MCC's long history as first-responders to the AIDS pandemic and called for a time of rebirth and restoration in that ongoing work. Members of Metropolitan Community Churches began to explore a number of ways to approach service and partnership with the incredible people "on the ground" in Africa, and a seed was planted that would grow at a steady, sustainable pace.

On Valentine's Day of 2006, MCCGHAM joined delegations from the Yvette A. Flunder Foundation, Refuge Ministries, and other partnered groups to visit the Mother of Peace Orphanage in rural Zimbabwe. We found a sacred community, first envisioned in a prophesy about the land and a special work there, and brought into being to offer succor and comfort to the children of Zimbabwe, to celebrate the power of faith in Christ and to welcome all who needed rest and healing.

Mother Jean and her sister, Mother Stella, both dedicated people of faith, pursued the prophetic vision to the site of a former lepers' colony on the side of a mountain known in the Shona language as *Mutemwa*, meaning "cut off." The women prayed, worked on the land, and allowed word to spread that they would help children in need — that no child living with or affected by HIV and AIDS would be turned away.

Overview of Chapter (continued)

Over time, children arrived from neighboring and distant villages, and the community grew. In each child, Mother Jean, Mother Stella and the people who had joined their mission saw the possibility of revitalization and resurrection for the people of Zimbabwe. They knew that if the children could be provided with good nutrition, clean water, medication and tender loving care, then with prayer and God's help they had a chance to make a difference.

Bishop Yvette Flunder and her partner, Mother Shirley Miller, guided the 2006 mission to the orphanage. With the help of Bishop Flunder's years of experience, wisdom and direction, MCCGHAM and our ministers began to build a relationship that would became a central focus of the ministry for 2006 and 2007. During our week in Zimbabwe that year, our hearts were blessed by the smiles and hugs of nearly 200 children. We surrendered to the touch of their tiny hands, and they shared their homes, their lives and their hope for life.

We in turn tried to offer our churches a glimpse into the children's lives. We shared travel journals and on World AIDS Day in 2006, sent out the DVD documentary, *We Who Are One Body: A Spiritual Walk With AIDS.* In our sermons and our presentations we told the story of the orphanage growing from a kernel of faith to a productive community, flourishing with abundant love for one another and the earnest pursuit of Jesus' example. Yes, they've suffered hardships along the way — 97 children are buried on the side of the mountain because medications were too scarce or treatment was begun too late — but the people of the community hold true to their cause.

During our 2006 stay at the orphanage, one of the tiny babies, Baby Anthony, passed away in the night. As is common in Africa, by the time he was brought into the orphanage, restoring the infant to full health was not physically possible — he was too far gone. The graves in the children's cemetery at the orphanage bear witness to almost a hundred stories like Anthony's. When a child dies all the members of the community stop what they are doing and gather to mourn the loss, honor the passage and celebrate the marriage of life and death. We were honored by the opportunity to share in Baby Anthony's funeral and to join in the prayers offered up on his behalf that day.

Over time the orphanage has been able to expand its mission. In addition to serving some 200 children, the staff operates a clinic which offers free medical care and support to the surrounding villages. The clinic's supply of medications is quite limited, but with the partnership of Dr. Robert Scott, from Oakland, California (USA) they have been able to offer direct care to a remarkable number of people in this rural region. During the 2007 trip, we served with the orphanage staff in the clinic while Dr. Scott saw more than 400 patients with AIDS, many of whom were also afflicted with tuberculosis and/or other serious illnesses.

And all the while we were there, the people of the orphanage sang. They sang to us when we arrived; they sang while they worked; they sang for fun, in celebration and in worship. The sounds of their voices joined together in hope and love never failed to lift our spirits and help us understand what it means to make a joyful noise. To sing praises to God and welcome to friends, both in the face of unrelenting adversity, is to possess and bestow a powerful spiritual gift.

A year has now passed since we last visited the Mother of Peace Orphanage and placed ourselves in the very heart of their mission, but the power of the experience to educate, awaken and inspire is undiminished. It still glows brightly and we will journey to join them again. In our contacts with Mother Jean — direct when she visited the United States and indirect through Bishop Flunder's team of dedicated ministers — she expresses continuing and deep gratitude to all the people of faith who help keep the mission alive. She and her sister, Stella, have committed their lives to God and to this work for as long as they are able to continue.

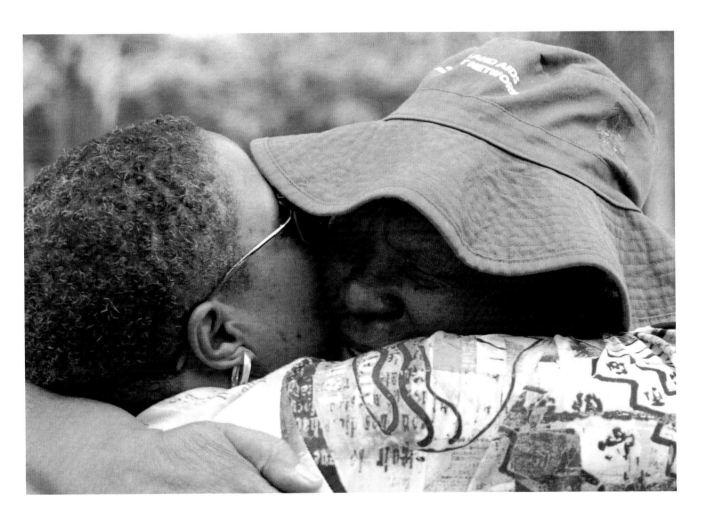

AGENDA FOR SESSION

Notes to the Facilitator
Room Set-Up
Full group discussion for the *Uncommon Hope* program works best in a circle if group size permits. If your meeting space will not accommodate such an arrangement, then angled rows from which participants can easily turn to see their peers in other seats will work. As you arrange your meeting space, consider accessibility issues in the event that you have differently-abled persons attending the sessions. It is very important to check on sound and noise levels to ensure that participants will be able to hear presentations as well as each other's comments and feedback. You may wish to break into pairs or small groups for parts of the discussion; if so, plan ahead for any movement of people or furniture. As much as possible, try to anticipate any physical accomodations your participants may need — larger print materials or the services of an ASL or BSL interpreter, for example.

Readings
It is recommended that participants have access to and read the journal entries reproduced in this chapter before they meet together for this session. The material can be copied from this facilitator's guide or downloaded from *www.UncommonHope.org* for email distribution.

Supplies
This session requires a copy of the previously mentioned journal entries for each participant, the DVD which accompanies the *Uncommon Hope* curriculum, a DVD player with connections to speakers and a playback screen (or screens) large enough to accommodate a screening for the entire group and journaling supplies for each participant. You may also want to have a large pad of paper or a whiteboard, appropriate markers and an easel.

If you are presenting this session as a stand-alone unit; that is, your participants have not already worked through some previous chapter or chapters, you will need to plan for introducing yourself as well as facilitating group introductions. Additionally, you will need to present the *Uncommon Hope* Group Guidelines as part of your introduction to the session. A sample introductory script and a copy of the guidelines begin on page 35 of this book. Be sure to insert the Chapter 6 title, "One Body: Gaining a Global Perspective" in place of the Chapter 1 title if you follow the Sample Script.

Session Length
The preferred session length is either 4 hours with a snack or meal break in the middle or two sessions of 2 hours each separated by no more than a week. Regardless of the session length you opt for, do plan on short, hourly breaks. If your session is structured to include a meal, assign small group discussion during that extended break. When people are beginning to know each other, some of the most exciting bonding and sharing can take place in the context of breaking bread together.

Welcome, Introduction of any New Participants and Warm-Up Exercises

Notes to the Facilitator

If you are presenting Chapter 6 as a stand-alone session, this is the point at which you should introduce yourself, facilitate the introduction of participants and read the Group Guidelines. If your participants have already worked through Chapter 1, a quick reminder of the Guidelines, particularly if you have been able to post them in your meeting space, should be sufficient.

Each session of *Uncommon Hope* offers participants the opportunity to explore their own spiritual lives more deeply and to connect more profoundly with others in the group. The process begins at an almost unconscious level when participants first enter the workshop space and becomes overt as individuals share their names a little more formally in the time set for Introductions. To further promote the transition from "outside lives" to the special time of group interaction, you should engage the group in a mindfully preparatory exercise at the beginning of each session. Each community may create its own introductory experiences or you may draw from the activities list provided in the Appendix.

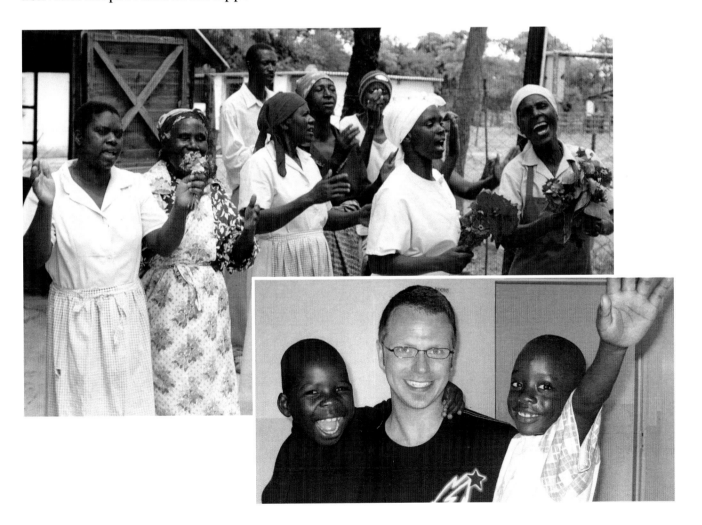

INTRODUCTION TO SESSION 6

In this session, participants are exposed to one example of expanding HIV and AIDS ministries into a global context. This is an opportunity for exploring partnerships with ministries already "on the ground" where the impacts of HIV and AIDS are most acutely felt right now. Powerful ministry is underway but there is an ongoing need for support. Through small group discussion of Joshua L. Love's Africa Trip journals and a large group viewing of the documentary *We Who Are One Body: a Spiritual Walk with AIDS*, participants can begin to envision taking sustainable actions that are global in nature yet still right-sized for their communities of faith.

SMALL GROUP EXERCISE

Have the participants read and discuss the following journal entries in small groups. (If every participant has pre-read and you have several strong readers in the group, it can be effective to do this reading aloud.) Suggest to the participants that their discussion after the reading should include, but not necessarily be limited to, their responses to these questions:

- **What kind of projects and efforts do you feel called to in the global response to HIV and AIDS?**
- **Are there ways your current HIV and AIDS efforts can connect to global efforts that are already in place?**
- **What impacts might unexamined racism, classism, colonialism, sexism, ageism, heterosexism, etc., have on your ministry efforts in a global context?**
- **How might awareness and understanding of different cultural styles of communication and community-building be important to your partnerships in global HIV and AIDS response?**
- **How can you work to create culturally-sensitive and culturally-appropriate partnerships with people living in contexts different from your own?**

The questions are reprinted after the journal entries.

MCCGHAM Trips to Mother of Peace Orphanage in Zimbabwe, Africa 2006 & 2007
Journal Entries (excerpts)
Joshua L. Love

2006 – Day 1 Reflection

As I write these words, I am sitting in the airport in Johannesburg, South Africa with an incredible delegation of faithful people. We are a multi-denominational, multi-racial and multi-generational group, and our individual experiences with HIV and AIDS range across a broad spectrum as well.

We all gathered in the United States to begin this journey together, and now, having arrived on the African continent, our collective excitement is all but palpable. The combination of seasoned travelers and first time visitors to Africa is making for a lovely balance.

We leave here in a few hours and fly to Zimbabwe. From the airport there, we'll travel by bus to meet the people who live at, operate, and support the services of the Mother of Peace Orphanage. Theirs is a specific mission to support children and adults living with and affected by HIV and AIDS. The orphanage was founded and is administered by Mother Jean and a loving, dedicated staff.

While we're at the orphanage, we'll spend time in service projects, respite for the workers, education and compassionate care for the residents. The orphanage strives for sustainability. They grow their own vegetables and fruit, tend a small collection of livestock and just last year built a dam for a fish farm.

The children love to have visitors and we are thrilled to go and learn about their lives.

> **As a person living with HIV, I consider this a sacred pilgrimage to a place at once familiar and completely unknown.**
> Rev. Elder Jim Mitulski

> **The struggle against Apartheid brought me to Africa the first time, the challenge of HIV brings me back.**
> Rev. G. Penny Nixon

It is important that those of us from the United States put our bodies and conscious minds in the very heart of this struggle.

This trip embodies the ethic of commitment to faithful service that all of us travelers pursue in our walks with one another and God.

2006 – Day 2 Reflection

Life comes and goes on the side of "Cut Off Mountain."

We lost Baby Anthony last night. He was around eleven months old and one of the "skeleton" babies we met yesterday. His tiny frame seemed barely large enough to hold a human spirit and was much too frail to continue suffering what he'd already experienced.

Anthony passed from the embrace of this community and into the hands of God in the deepest night. Several of our group held him yesterday afternoon – supported him physically and repeatedly spoke messages of deep love and care. Mother Jean, the faithful matriarch of this community, grieved him quietly through the day. The orphanage and clinic teams worked so very hard to give him the chance to keep living after he came to stay.

Many of us have already developed a strong emotional tie to these children. It is impossible to feel hardened when you're exposed to their love. Even Baby Anthony, who we knew so briefly, taught us to use every possible second to connect and care...there are no guarantees that more moments will follow.

Early this morning we wandered sleepily to our work duties. The Mother of Peace staff has graciously allowed us to fit ourselves into their well-developed routines. Some of us headed to the clinic; others are serving at the preschool or on the farm.

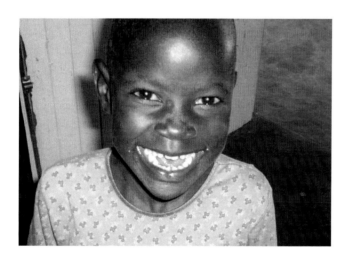 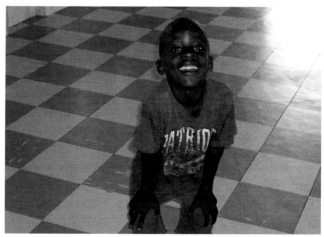

Dr. Scott asked Rev. Elder Jim Mitulski and me to come to the clinic and offer HIV prevention counseling. We arrived at around 7:45 AM to find a line out the door and snaking across much of the clinic's lawn. Some 400-500 people had come, some walking as far as 40 or 50 km, to wait in line for any kind of treatment!

Other members of our group were already assisting the doctor and his staff with the first patients. In order to be seen the people had to have brought a medical treatment card, which I thought looked like an elementary school student's notebook. Cardholders were provided with whatever medication they needed until the "tablets" ran out.

Dr. Scott's nurse, David, took Rev. Elder Mitulski and me back to an unfinished portion of the clinic. The volunteers set us up in simple concrete rooms with a couple of chairs and some condoms, and offered some remarkably short instructions before leaving us there. We were told that the majority of the people we were about to see would be HIV-positive or in a family with someone who was HIV-positive, and we were told that each session would last from 5 to 7 minutes.

A translator was assigned to each of us — we were paired with young men from a large city in Zimbabwe who had come to orphanage specifically to aid our group's efforts. Their support proved to be incredibly valuable in conversation after difficult conversation.

We were behind before we even began. The time estimates for each conversation were entirely too short. Many of the people we saw had never been to the clinic before and had arrived without knowing whether or not the doctor would even be able to see them. We saw young people, older people, people who seemed fit and strong, and people whose symptoms seemed obvious to even our untrained eyes. There was no way for us to know before a person walked in the door what care he or she might need.

While it was at times productive to talk about HIV transmission and the need for protection, most of the people we saw came with complex medical problems well beyond our capacity or the scope of our simple mission. In the first hour alone, we talked with HIV-positive widows, heterosexual couples, both whom were HIV-positive, single men and women, children, and a number of people diagnosed with tuberculosis or other diseases *in addition to* HIV! The conditions these people faced — economically and medically — were staggering. Many had no food to eat, had received no prior care for their HIV and despaired of their chances for survival. But still they were desperate for help, and they lined up in the early morning and waited for hours to be seen because of their deep, passionate desire for help.

Married women were clearly disadvantaged in their control over their own bodies. Most articulated that their husbands held the authority to insist on having sex without condoms — they were, after all, legal wives. One unmarried woman, who worked in local HIV prevention, told me that it was better to be a man's mistress than his wife because a mistress can insist on condoms, but a wife cannot.

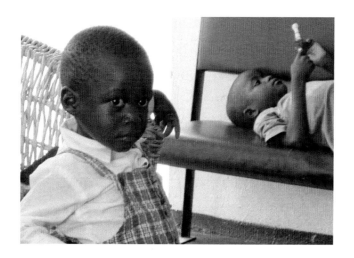
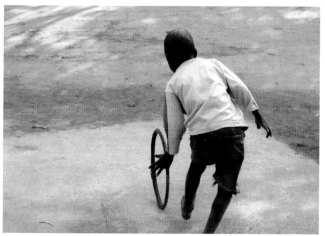

The men rarely offered direct information when we asked how they'd been exposed to HIV. For example, one man shared that he had been married for 17 years to the same woman and that they had 4 children ranging in age from 2 to 15 years. Both he and his wife tested HIV-positive within the last year and neither has received any medication or treatment. The man never mentioned having had other sexual partners, and over and over throughout the day, other men told stories which contained the same silent implication.

Many of the patients we saw expressed shame about revealing their HIV-positive status to their loved ones, especially parents with children. There existed a widespread belief that family members would be adversely affected by the knowledge that HIV had entered their home life. Some of the people living with the virus feared being rejected by family and friends, losing a job, or being treated badly in their communities. Those fears felt very familiar — our experience in the United States has been much the same.

Every visit required a near-instant assessment and decision about what approach to take and what level of information to offer. I revealed my own HIV-positive status to one of the first few groups and Pride, my translator, relayed the information about my status and my multi-year survival with the virus. Next door, Rev. Elder Mitulski shared his story of long-term survival and outside, under the trees where she had begun to see patients, Rev. Nixon spoke about her positive friends and parishioners. These revelations, so common in all of our daily lives, shocked many of the patients. One woman gasped and said to me, "But you are so fit." A young boy touched Rev. Elder Mitulski and said, "Belly" with a sense of wonder at his apparent health.

We faced the complex variances in our own cultural and physical experience of HIV and AIDS. The inequities and the difference between AIDS experiences in United States and Zimbabwe emerged on many unexpected levels. It was, at first, easy to feel advantaged by our access to medications and economic resources, more than 10 years "post-protease." For both Rev. Elder Mitulski and myself, he a long-term survivor and me close behind, the tendency to see HIV as a multi-year survival process rather than a death sentence was suddenly highlighted. The circumstance created an immediate sense of the healthy "haves" of the United States of America and the systemically poor "have nots" of the vulnerable communities we were encountering.

It was one of the most ethically and emotionally challenging experiences we could have imagined. When we talked in a small group later, we reflected that while we had access to medicines and economic stability, the people of Zimbabwe we had encountered had a fierce determination to live. None of the men and women we met with was being treated for depression. We saw no complicit turns to nihilism nor any of the self-destructive behavior that we see all too frequently in our own communities. We began to see that there were no "haves" and "have nots" but rather a multitude of lenses through which to experience HIV and AIDS. Length of life... the hope for more life...perhaps it is in the grappling to understand what to do next when you find yourself HIV-positive that we come closest to a universal focus.

The day passed at an exhausting pace. The line of patients never seemed to shorten; the need never waned. The complex spiritual and psychic pain of these lives took our breath away.

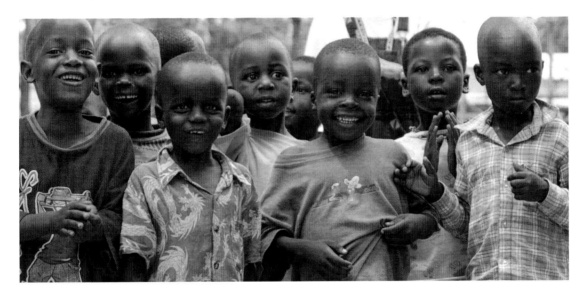

In the middle of the day, we paused to eat a little food and join the funeral service for Baby Anthony. The children banged a metal disc outside the chapel as a call to the community to attend the passage of one of their own. It was one of the most grace-filled funerals I have ever witnessed. Preschool children, in hushed respect, filled the floor of the chapel and the staff streamed in from all the invisible corners of the grounds. We all sat where we could and were lovingly welcomed. The gathered people sang until the tiny coffin entered the chapel and then we all stood in reverential silence. Catholic prayers and scriptures were read aloud in the local language — an inspired and inspiring marriage of cultures and respect.

The coffin was then lifted and the next part of Anthony's passage was begun. Dr. Scott took the coffin in his arms and the entire population – children and adults, women and men, residents and visitors alike – followed him to the children's cemetery. Small children, in almost total silence, drifted to the adults. They chose us and took our hands, sometimes several children clustered around a single adult. There was a simple grace to the ritual and as the children held our hands, guiding us down the dusty path, they taught us how to hold Baby Anthony in our hearts.

When we got to the rough grass near the edge of the cemetery, they paused and tugged our hands. No instructions were given, but we understood and the children climbed up to be carried, like Anthony, the last bit of the way – the living and the dead in accord.

The same holy woman who presided over the chapel service spoke over the open grave. She led us through scripture and prayer, consecrated the grave with holy water, and then the men laid the tiny coffin into the ground. The women of the community, accompanied by gentle drumbeats, sang to Anthony, and the men took up shovels and rocks and gently closed the grave.

To complete the ceremony, Mother Jean drew all of the little children to the small, newly-raised mound, and they planted flowers and small plants collected from all around the farm. When they were done, each child returned to his or her chosen adult and they led us back across the grass to the next part of our day.

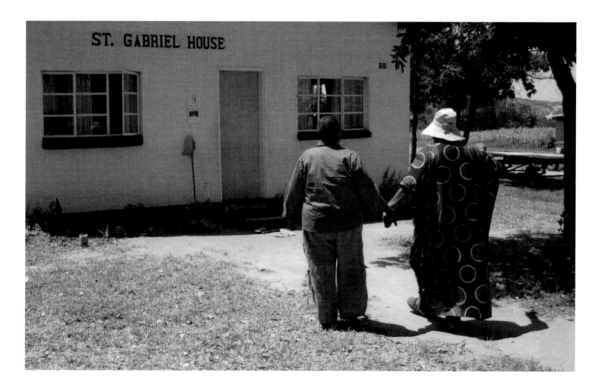

The afternoon sessions were even longer than those of the morning. Everyone at the clinic met people one after another, with virtually no break until nearly 7 PM. The backlog of patients grew until we had to start taking them in groups of three and four at a time. More people came from the surrounding communities and at some point, though we weren't aware of exactly when, someone on the other side of the clinic had to begin making hard decisions about turning people away.

In our talks after dark, we noted that we arrived in Zimbabwe in the "protease moment" akin to what we'd experienced in the U.S. in 1995. Many more of these people will die before the medications have a real and lasting effect — the history of HIV told in other cemeteries on another continent. These children and their parents will die not because efficacious drugs don't exist but because they weren't made available in this economically challenged country.

The "Baby Anthonys" of Zimbabwe are passing in the middle of the night because help is coming too late.

There is still so much work to do.

2006 – Day 3 Reflection

The emotional impact of the time we spent at the clinic yesterday weighs heavily on all our minds, hearts, and spirits. Rev. Nixon went over first thing this morning to help with the last group of patients Dr. Scott will see before he leaves for the city, (where he will see even more HIV patients.) The need for medical treatment exceeds the resources of the clinic. People will have to be sent home, and some will die because they have no "tablets," food or shelter.

No matter how many times we talk it through and try to come to terms with this situation, it continues to overwhelm our emotions. There is so little we can do in the limited time we have here.

The rest of the day has been allocated to casual time with the children.

Rev. Elder Mitulski describes the community here as being similar to an abbey of the Middle Ages. Mother Jean acts as the Abbess and with her sisters and workers, she has created a small village of inter-dependent care.

We took time in the afternoon to sit with Mother Jean and listen to the history of her work. She told us the story of how a woman prophesied about "Cut Off Mountain" — that the land on the side of the mountain would become the home of a holy community built around "7 Cares":

1. Care for the disabled
2. Care for the terminally ill
3. Care for the caregiver
4. Care for the spiritually ill
5. Care for finances — self-sufficiency
6. Care for God's bounty — the land
7. Care for the new order — an inclusive community

Each of these "Cares" would direct the community's actions to continuing the work of Christ. They were to serve children, worship God, and prepare the way for the Second Coming.

The self-assured way in which she shared these stories made each layer seem clearer than the last. We talked for a couple of hours with Mother Jean about how they built this thriving community from a patch of unwanted land. It was an incredible and tender story of faith and commitment.

In the beginning, there was nothing in this place but thorny trees and brush. Mother Jean came to the area with a small handful of people and they looked for ways to be useful. They cleared and piled rocks for later use, laid down paths and the mission began to grow literally from the ground up. Mother Jean laughs when she thinks back to those first four years in a trailer. Her joy at God's blessings to her family and the children of the orphanage overflows and touches each of us.

She says they knew that the prophecy had been valid when the children began to arrive. The first child turned up in 1995 — an infant with hands and feet all turned in, who the mission hospital doctors didn't expect to live for more than 6 or 7 months. The child survived for almost two years with Mother Jean and her group pouring their love into the tiny body and spirit. The second child was HIV-positive upon arrival in 1996, but tested HIV-negative two years later. By the end of 1996 there were 6 children with Mother Jean and her group, and word was spreading in the surrounding communities that there was a place for the orphans.

People asked Mother Jean why they took in the AIDS orphans. She explained that they took in children who lost their parents to accidents, disease, all sorts of causes — the children were simply orphans not "AIDS orphans." Further, if no other orphanage in the region would care for children orphaned by AIDS, many of them also HIV-positive, then Mother of Peace would take them and make a place for them.

The children's individual stories rearrange the internal landscapes of our hearts. Gerald, Manuel, Spence, Tanai, Moses, Emanuel, Joseph, Veronika, Cephas, Jeremiah, Vincent, Casper, Hilda, Peter, Michele, Nyasha, Pheneas, Chido, Ventu and so many more are the living inheritors of the prophesy.

Anthony, Memory, Patrick, David, Perpetua, Gift, Petronela and dozens of others did not live long lives but their brief journeys are no less important to the manifestation of this mission. God called them home and calls us to witness their lives and hold up the accomplishments of their short lives: these babies, children and teens survived just long enough to open the hearts of their caretakers. Like pebbles splashing into a pond, they made an impact which spread into the local villages and eventually across the ocean to all of us.

Halfway around the world, Bishop Flunder felt the call to serve the community centered about the orphanage. Her visits to Africa inform the work she does in the United States. She shares the stories of the children at Mother of Peace with all the communities she touches, and those stories serve as guideposts to greater healing and movement.

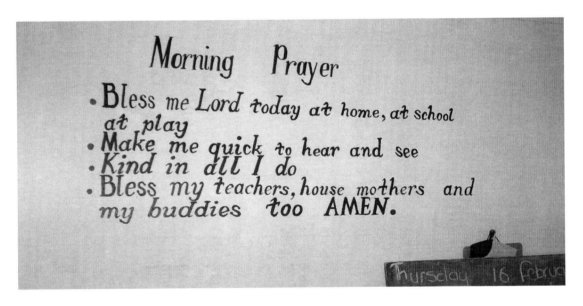

Bishop Flunder reached out to Metropolitan Community Churches and a new joint mission to support the work of Mother of Peace began. One of the most glaringly obvious needs of our time is the commitment to work in tandem and in sustained support of project-based ministries.

By the end of the third day, Dr. Scott has left the orphanage. We are filled with stories and shared moments. The children wander in and out and move freely amongst us. Some of the members of our group are beginning to have questions about our own accountability.

The greatest eye-opener of this trip has been the recognition that I have received far more than I could have given, learned more than I taught and grown beyond my most extreme hopes. As far I am concerned, Mother of Peace has offered "care to the caregiver."

Zimbabwe sings to us. Cries in the night call us out of our laziness, then we wake to drumbeats and joyful songs. The singers soothe and heal with their peaceful and passionate lyrics. We are aware of a sense of overflowing happiness at the collective music and rhythms of life God has called into being here.

The power of this day, for me at least, is that I'm still being changed. After yesterday, I was certain I had no reserves left to be wrung out...and then today came. A child smiled. A spiritual leader told me a story. I caught a song in my heart and I discovered another small lesson God had hidden away inside me.

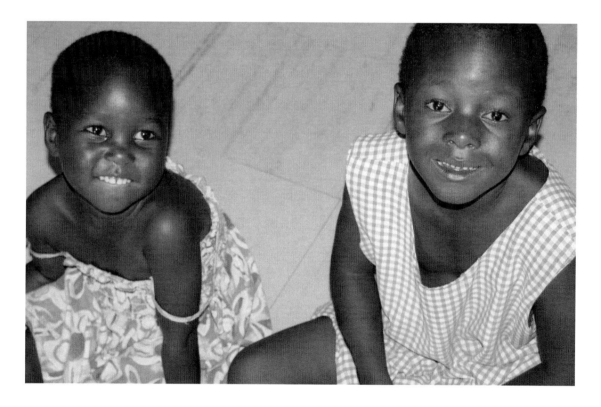

2007 – Day 2 Reflection

Our flight from London to Harare provided some time for gentle reflection. I remembered the faces of the children, the painful loss of Baby Anthony, the struggle of the people who walked for miles to visit the clinic and be seen by Doctor Scott, and most of all the passion and love of Mother Jean and Mother Stella, who keep the heart of this mission intact.

We arrived early Wednesday morning and were greeted by friends we'd met last year. We spent the day resting from the trip, overcoming jetlag and orienting new members of the delegation to this exciting experience.

The cool of the evening came gently upon us as we gathered for our first group meal. We sat together to break bread and share fellowship. While some of our talk focused on our work or old times, there was another persistent theme: our universal anticipation of the presence of God at the orphanage and our respect for the hard work being done here. Bishop Flunder brought us into a place of laughter and accountability in her special way.

We went our separate ways after dinner and lay down to sleep, each with anticipation of the spiritual walk ahead. For some of us, tomorrow morning will be a time of reunion, for some a time of pilgrimage, for some a moment of rest and for some a time of rebirth. The individual threads of our experiences begin to weave together to create a strong cloth...a fabric of the spirit.

2007 – Day 3 Report

> **"O Mwari wangu ndinotendera ndinovimba, ndinokurumbidzai nokukudai. Ndinokumbira ruregerero kuna avo vasingatenderi vasinga vimbi nemi nevasingakudei. Amen."**
> prayer of the children at the orphanage

A flat, rusty metal disc hangs outside the chapel, a material focal point. From this central point at the very heart of the community, the paths connecting the physical structures of this place — the houses, the clinic, the newly built skills center and several other buildings — spiral out. Faith and prayer inhabit the spiritual core and radiate outward to infuse each of the structures and the lives within them.

The clanging of that metal gong calls the children and workers to assemble for worship and to bear witness to God. Twice during our stay the call sounded for a late afternoon Rosary service. Mother Stella, a woman whose life was reconstructed by her relationship to the Creator, holds the space for these times of reflection and prayer. She enters the chapel ahead of the little ones and as they enter, she guides them into reverent, kneeling rows. The breeze blows in through the open windows and a gentle peace washes through the place of worship. Later, Rev. Elder Glenna Shepherd observed, "The children come to worship of their own initiative. They enter the chapel and eagerly head for the baptismal waters, placing the sign of the cross on their bodies. I had a sense that worship was as much a part of life as eating or sleeping — done with joy, peace and fullness."

In their native language, the children recite the prayers of the Rosary, the older children rarely missing a word while the youngest look on and are instructed by their intent observation. Young voices lead each section of prayer. Mother Stella speaks above them from time to time but only to make minor corrections. Occasionally eyelids droop and a small head begins to nod. Mother Stella reaches out with a gentle touch or rises to collect the weary ones and bring them close to her to help keep them alert. I saw only one boy whose nap went unnoticed — he sat almost straight up and just a hint of a sway betrayed his true state.

The rhythm of the "Hail Mary" feels familiar even though the prayer is rendered in the local language. I cannot distinguish some of the other prayers as readily, but I can make educated guesses by watching the slow pull of the rosary beads through the palm of a nearby prayer leader. Every few sections a prayer is repeated in English, "Oh my God, I believe, I trust, I adore and I love you, and I beg pardon for those who do not believe, who do not adore, who do not trust, and who do not love you. Amen." Near the end of the period of reflection the children rise and lift their voices. Drums provide support for their songs and a few of the youngsters engage in a dance of adoration and celebration. Their knees bend slightly and their arms reach out, one forward one to the rear, to scissor up and down.

In both services, tears come to my eyes. These children, in the care of powerful women who live by faith, are learning the rituals and practice of their faith tradition. The gift they are receiving shines in many of their eyes. Blessings are abundant here, freely given and easily accepted.

2007 – Day 4 Report – Morning/Afternoon

After breakfast, Mother Jean and Mother Stella walk the short path to the chapel with a few of us. On each of my visits to the orphanage I collect images and video that will, with God's help, open a door between our churches and this holy place. Recording people's intimate thoughts and narratives and attempting to translate those experiences to our beloved communities around the world constitutes a sacred trust. I consider receiving and sharing the words and ideas these generous souls entrust to my care to be an act of prayer.

Mothers Jean and Stella breathe a touch of order, a liberal measure of compassion and a lion's share of love into the lives of all who pass through their gates. The two women have hundreds of bodies and souls in their direct care, and their reach extends exponentially as they pass resources into the surrounding community by employing many part-time workers, feeding volunteers, trading agricultural and farm goods, and providing a clinic for HIV and AIDS care in partnership with Dr. Scott.

When I ask Mother Jean to tell me stories about individual members of her constructed family, she details their life walks in frank terms. Many of her stories begin with an account of the pain or loss that brought the individual, often a child, to Mother of Peace. She then she proceeds to relate the particulars of how good nutrition, tender loving care, medication, and most importantly prayer were incorporated and applied in each case.

Each story follows its own unique track. Lives lost have a presence in both Mother Jean's and Mother Stella's memories; so, too, do many amazing sagas of restoration and survival. Many of the stories they call forward are still in progress and are girded about with surpassing hope. As I listen, ears keen to capture every bit they offer, I begin to understand that my story sits in their care now, too, along with the stories of the many people who have become Spirit-connected to this place and these powerful women.

Two events stirred intense emotions within the first 36 hours of last year's pilgrimage. First, Baby Anthony, the eleven-month-old who we held and kissed and prayed over, passed in the middle of the night. Second, Dr. Scott opened the doors of the on-site clinic to a group of some 400 to 500 people who had arrived by foot hoping desperately to receive something to help them survive. That clinic now operates briefly every three months to provide medical care and anti-retroviral medications to the people of the orphanage and the surrounding communities.

Experiencing the intersection of the baby's death and the clinic's birth was profoundly cathartic and shook me deeply. Rather than feeling distanced by the myriad differences between our lives and the lives of the people in this rural community, I found my heart beating very near to theirs. My thoughts and feelings and the reactions rising and falling within me were realigned during our shared hours and the new patterns will carry forward. My story shifted along fault lines I didn't even know were there, and I cracked open to make room in my heart to carry Baby Anthony and the people of the clinic next to my own history. I could actually feel the expansion happening. In some way, I imagine I'll continue to feel it for a long time.

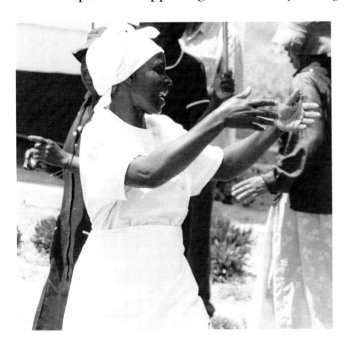 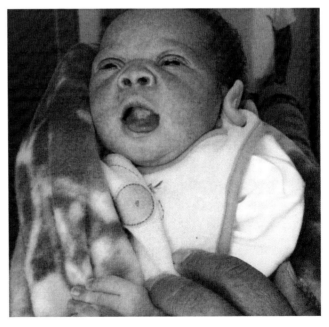

2007 – Day 4 Report – Evening

As I did last year, I am again experiencing a feeling of my spirit settling into a comfortable and comforting natural rhythm. I have been shooting video and pictures with Christy Ebner (MCCGHAM Program Assistant,) touring the houses the children live in, visiting the primary school, processing the stories we collect and visiting the dam and the children's cemetery. Even with all of that activity, God has made room for sit-down meals with long talks, tears and laughter.

Time at the orphanage seems to move differently – so unlike the rapid-fire pace of our lives back home. It almost as if each day is somehow expanded by an extra measure of hours. I suppose that's because in this place we operate on spiritual rather than linear time.

Rev. Elder Shepherd says, "The rhythms of nature and the in-the-moment attention that the children elicit from us puts time right somehow. Living in the moment in this place makes me more aware of my feelings, makes spaces for reflection, and offers me deep rest when the day ends."

In the presence of these children and the adults who raise and protect them, the concept of legacy emerges. There are, to be sure, kaleidoscopic variations on the theme of legacy – organic, instructional, spiritual and physical – but it is clear that information, culture, survival skills and love are passed on, from generation to generation. With God and Mother Jean set at a spiritual and ancestral axis, this growth and "passing on" radiates outward through the community. Mother Stella, Mother Jean's sister, younger by 16 years, followed her into this calling. Men and women of the community have come here, been touched and changed, and have carried that spiritual healing and heritage into their own families.

As visitors with a commitment to partnership, all of us from the several delegations, have come to receive instruction and wisdom from these teachers, so we can return home to teach others and return with resources to better serve the children at the orphanage. We are becoming a part of the legacy as well as contributing to its process.

Perhaps because of the presence of children, with their straightforward, almost unconscious access to the sacred, my perception of "legacy" seems both wider and more immediate. As a person living with HIV in my body, I have struggled with an occasional thought that all the accumulated wisdom and strength that has been shared so generously with me will be lost if I don't stay healthy enough to raise children of my own. Yet here with small, sticky hands clutching me and the wizened eyes of Mother Jean looking into mine, I see that those passages, the legacies we carry, are not based on time or genetics. Each moment of relationship is an opportunity to pass on a bit of what we carry.

Bishop Flunder has said that she learns a lot about power and love just by watching Mother Jean and Mother Stella. She watches them moving through the changing tides of their lives with God and receives a deeper knowing. The orphanage holds the seeds of many new starts, of many moments that will repair the world, of many hopes and of the collective history of God's people. Perhaps holding that sacred trust is part of what legacy is really about.

The journal entries end here but the story, of course, continues.

In a small group (or groups) share your reactions and responses to the journal entries you've read. Your discussion should include, but not necessarily be limited to, consideration of the following questions:

- What kind of projects and efforts do you feel called to in the global response to HIV and AIDS?
- Are there ways your current HIV and AIDS efforts can connect to global efforts that are already in place?
- What impacts might unexamined racism, classism, colonialism, sexism, ageism, heterosexism, etc., have on your ministry efforts in a global context?
- How might awareness and understanding of different cultural styles of communication and community-building be important to your partnerships in global HIV and AIDS response?
- How can you work to create culturally-sensitive and culturally-appropriate partnerships with people living in contexts different from your own?

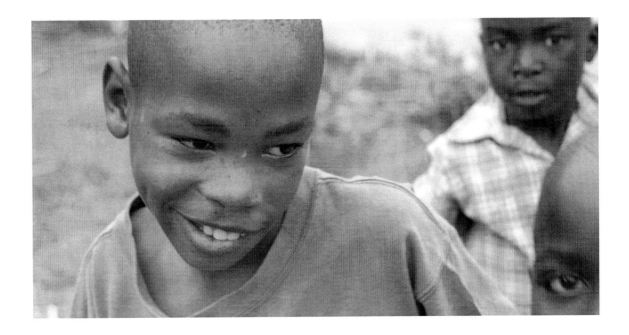

LARGE GROUP EXERCISE

View the documentary film *We Who Are One Body: A Spiritual Walk With AIDS.* Discuss your reactions and responses.

Notes to the Facilitator

If possible, allow the participants some time for individual reflection before initiating the large group discussion. As the large group discusses the film and their responses to it, encourage participants to include and incorporate any related elements from their small group discussions about the journal entries.

CLOSING MEDITATION/POEM/PRAYER/RITUAL/SONG

Note to the Facilitator

This can be created by the participants or drawn from any resource that is compatible with the faith traditions represented in the group.

Closing Meditation

> What actions are most excellent?
> To gladden the heart of a human being.
> To feed the hungry.
> To help the afflicted.
> To lighten the sorrow of the sorrowful.
> To remove the wrongs of the injured.
> That person is the most beloved of God
> who does most good to God's creatures.

The Prophet Mohammad

I must confess that I have enjoyed being on this mountaintop and I am tempted to want to stay here and retreat to a more quiet and serene life. But something within reminds me that the valley calls me in spite of all its agonies, dangers, and frustrating moments. I must return to the valley. Something tells me that the ultimate test of a man is not where he stands in moments of comfort and moments of convenience, but where he stands in moments of challenge and moments of controversy.

Rev. Dr. Martin Luther King, Jr., 1965

All of us have been given to drink of one Spirit. And that Body is not one part; it is many. If the foot should say, "Because I am not a hand, I do not belong to the body," does that make it any less a part of the body? If the ear should say, "Because I am not an eye, I do not belong to the body," would that make it any less a part of the body? If the body were all eye, what would happen to the hearing? If it were all ear, what would happen to the sense of smell? Instead of that God put all the parts into one body on purpose. If all the parts were alike, what would the body be? They are, indeed, many different members but one body. They eye cannot say to the hand, "I do not need you," anymore than the head can say to the feet, "I do not need you." And even those members which seem less important are in fact indispensible. We honor the members we consider less honorable by clothing them with greater care, thus bestowing on the less presentable a propriety which the more presentable do not need. God has so constructed the body as to give greater honor to the lowly members, that there may be no dissension among the body, but that all of the members may be concerned for one another. If one member suffers, all the members suffer with it; if one member is honored, all the members share its joy.

1 Corinthian 12:14-26
*(*The Inclusive New Testament*, Priests for Equality, Brentwood MD, 1994)*

Chapter 6 Questions:

1. What sorts of projects and efforts do you feel called to in the global response to HIV and AIDS?

2. How might awareness and understanding of different cultural styles of communication and community-building be important to your partnership in global HIV and AIDS response?

3. How can you work to create culturally-sensitive and culturally-appropriate partnerships with people living in contexts different from your own?

4. In what ways has your personal call to HIV and AIDS service been impacted by your learning?

Chapter 6 Notes:

Conclusion

Things will always break apart and come together. Yet, in our pain, we often lose sight of their transformative connection: that each cocoon must break so the next butterfly can be. And it is our curse and blessing to die and be born so many times. So many sheddings. So many wings. But in this is the chief work of love: to comfort each other each time we break, to midwife each other each time we're born, and to be the missing piece in what we need to learn, again and again.

Mark Nepo, *The Exquisite Risk*, 2005

Nothing's lost forever. In this world, there's a kind of painful progress. Longing for what we've left behind, and dreaming ahead. At least I think that's so.

the character Harper Pitt in
Tony Kushner's *Angels in America*, 1991

Let all the fragmented parts of my being gather around You, help me to face them one by one. Love's healing presence will mend all that has been broken; I shall once again be made whole.

excerpt from Psalm 7 in
Nan C. Merrill's *Psalms for Praying*, 1997

Our exploration of the impact of HIV and AIDS in *Uncommon Hope* has taken us on a special pilgrimage of the spirit. Together we have journeyed through the immensity of loss, the magnitude of individual courage and the dangers of silence. At this point along our path, we can say unequivocally that, "Millions of lives and millions of deaths around the world bear direct witness to the fact that AIDS IS NOT OVER," and that our intentional work together is more necessary than ever.

- How will you show compassion to the people living with and affected by HIV and AIDS?
- How will you break the systems of silence, oppression and marginalization within which new infections continue to occur?
- How will you ensure that people living with and affected by HIV and AIDS are not separated from the Divine by human stigmatization and shame?
- What will you do to bring about the changes necessary in our shared world to bring an end to HIV and AIDS?

In response to these questions, some individuals will become activists and teachers. Others will recognize the negative impact their prejudices have had on vulnerable people, and will focus on healing, corrective action. Some may choose to engage in raising awareness within their local communities while others may feel personally called to partner with people in other parts of the world to create change. Some individuals will speak aloud the truth of their own life experiences as a persons living with and affected by HIV and AIDS, and in doing so help free people trapped in the silence born of stigmatization.

In short, this work is no more uniform than are our unique life experiences. The Divine has gifted us with a rich diversity and through it an almost endless capacity to respond creatively to adversity and challenge in our lives. Each of us has come this far along the road because we felt that healing was possible — that hope could yet live.

Our tasks now are as follows:
- To keep alive the lessons we have learned by passing them on
- To listen carefully to the real experiences of people living with HIV and AIDS
- To dismantle the systems of oppression which continue to make certain people inequitably vulnerable to new HIV infections
- To challenge the systems of power and privilege that do not yet afford adequate medical, spiritual, institutional and educational care to all people either vulnerable to HIV infection or already living with and affected by HIV and AIDS

We have met in *Uncommon Hope* and made a good beginning. Now together, we can look into each others' eyes with surety of purpose and say, "You are the *Uncommon Hope* of the future. You are the story yet to be told. You are, in fact, the end of AIDS."

Appendix

The activities described here may be used "as is" or adapted to suit the needs and preferences of your group of Uncommon Hope *participants. They are listed in no particular order and are included as resource materials rather than particularly recommended exercises.*

Crossing Truths

In this exercise the facilitator asks a number of questions, some of a trivial nature and others about weightier matters. The participants respond physically and with simple, direct movements begin to share something of themselves with each other.

To preface the activity, create an obstruction-free space within your meeting room and group all the participants on one side of that space. Tell the participants that you'll be asking yes/no questions and that they are to respond non-verbally by crossing the room whenever their answer is "Yes." Advise them that anyone may choose not to answer by simply remaining stationary. (Moving means "yes" but not moving doesn't necessarily mean "no.") Also tell them that they can cross the room incompletely – stop in the middle – to indicate either uncertainty or that a true answer would require some explanation.

Sample Questions:

1. Were you born in the southern United States?

2. Do you have siblings?

3. Have you ever been in a committed relationship?

4. Do you consider yourself to be a spiritual person?

5. Do you enjoy trying new foods?

6. Do you identify yourself as male (or female)?

7. Did you enjoy playing outside when you were a child?

8. Have you ever experienced racism?

9. Have you ever traveled to another country?

10. Do you consider yourself politically active?

11. Do you identify as transgender?

12. Have you ever considered yourself an activist in a cause that matters to you?

13. Do you enjoy musical theater (or opera or drag races or the symphony or...)?

14. Do you know someone living with HIV and/or AIDS?

Pause after each question to allow participants to respond and observe each other's responses, and then invite them to reassemble in one location before presenting the next question. Do remind the group members at least once that they may choose not to answer by remaining still and that they can respond equivocally by making an incomplete crossover.

This exercise does not need to take a very long time: 20 to 30 questions can be answered in a surprisingly short period. If the group is responding well and seems particularly engaged in finding out about each other, it may be productive to let them shout out their own questions. If you proceed this way, be certain that you monitor any extemporaneous questions for safety — this is an introductory exercise and the group should not be allowed to move into emotionally complex situations at this point.

We Remember
In this exercise participants test their knowledge of the history of HIV and AIDS. [It is recommended that you not pair this exercise with Chapter 1.] Prepare for this exercise by posting large sheets of paper showing a timeline with only the years between public recognition of AIDS the present labeled, and by writing key events in the history of HIV and AIDS on individual note cards.

Distribute the note cards randomly (shuffle and deal or allow participants to draw) and once each participant has at least one "event" in hand, encourage them to create an accurate chronology by affixing their card(s) — use tape — to the timeline. Suggest that participants work individually for several minutes but then encourage discussion and collaboration after they've made tentative placements.

Once all of the events are placed, check the order of the completed timeline. Support the group's learning by praising success as appropriate and making gentle corrections if needed. It is critically important that you, the facilitator, know or have ready access to the correct order of events; however, depending on the make-up of your group, you may find that allowing a few individuals to share brief memories will help the group "fix" the chronology. Do bear in mind that the collective remembrance, rather than the personal story, should be the primary focus at this time.

Who Said It?

Learning about the public statements that have been made about HIV and AIDS can help participants to feel the impact of public discourse on people living with HIV and AIDS. The words and comments of any number of people – celebrities, scientists, politicians, religious leaders and ordinary citizens – the famous, the infamous and the obscure – can be found with relative ease using simple internet searches.

For this activity select a variety of quotes about HIV and/or AIDS, then print or write out each statement and its speaker on separate sheets of paper. Distribute the papers randomly, making sure that each person in the room has at least one quote or one name, and then explain to the group members that they must match each quote with the person who said it.

Invite the participants to move about searching for the "mate" to their pieces of paper – you may allow them to organize their matching at will or you may suggest that they use wall space or table space to work out the correspondences. Once the participants are satisfied that they've arranged correct matches, review their work by speaking each quote aloud and identifying the speaker. [The educational value of this exercise can be enhanced by framing each statement in its original context – the facilitator must be well-prepared in order to provide that level of feedback for the participants. Alternately, the group may enjoy doing context research as an "outside" activity.]

Sample Quotes:

1. "It is bad enough that people are dying of AIDS, but no one should die of ignorance."
   Elizabeth Taylor, actress and activist who co-founded the American Foundation for AIDS Research (amfAR)

2. "AIDS is no longer a death sentence for those who can get the medicines. Now it's up to the politicians to create the 'comprehensive strategies' to better treat the disease."
   President Bill Clinton

3. "In today's climate in our country, which is sickened with the pollution of pollution, threatened with the prominence of AIDS, riddled with burgeoning racism, rife with growing huddles of the homeless, we need art and we need art in all forms. We need all methods of art to be present, everywhere present, and all the time present."
   Maya Angelou, author

4. "I have learned more about love, selflessness and human understanding in this great adventure in the world of AIDS than I ever did in the cut-throat, competitive world in which I spent my life."
   Anthony Perkins, actor

5. "HIV does not make people dangerous to know, so you can shake their hands and give them a hug: Heaven knows they need it."
   Diana, Princess of Wales

6. "The important thing is this: just because I'm doing well doesn't mean that they're going to do well if they get HIV. A lot of people have died since I have announced. This disease is not going anywhere."

Magic Johnson, former professional basketball player and HIV-positive man

7. "History will judge us on how we respond to the AIDS emergency in Africa....whether we stood around with watering cans and watched while a whole continent burst into flames....or not."

Bono, lead singer of the rock group U2

8. "AIDS destroys families, decimates communities and, particularly in the poorest areas of the world, threatens to destabilize the social, cultural, and economic fabric of entire nations..."

Rabbi David Saperstein, Director of the Religious Action Center of Reform Judaism

9. "The global HIV/AIDS epidemic is an unprecedented crisis that requires an unprecedented response. In particular it requires solidarity — between the healthy and the sick, between rich and poor, and above all, between richer and poorer nations. We have 30 million orphans already. How many more do we have to get, to wake up?"

Kofi Annan, General Secretary of the United Nations

10. "We are all sick because of AIDS, and we are all tested by this crisis. It is a test not only of our willingness to respond, but of our ability to look past the artificial divisions and debates that have often shaped that response. When you go to places like Africa and you see this problem up close, you realize that it's not a question of either treatment or prevention — or even what kind of prevention — it is all of the above. It is not an issue of either science or values — it is both. Yes, there must be more money spent on this disease. But there must also be a change in hearts and minds; in cultures and attitudes. Neither philanthropist nor scientist; neither government nor — church, can solve this problem on their own — AIDS must be an all-hands-on-deck effort."

Illinois Senator Barack Obama, World AIDS Day 2006

Remember My Name

This activity engages participants in creating descriptive names for themselves and sharing those names with the group in a cumulative, sequential process. [If/when you opt for this exercise, you should delay the creation of any name tags until after your group completes the activity.]

Arrange the participants, either sitting or standing, in a loose circle so that each of them can see all of the others' faces. Announce that each person is to think of a self-descriptive word that begins with the same letter as the name he or she prefers to use (i.e. Magical Marty, Creative Chris, Sassy Sandy, Boisterous BJ, Tall Terry, etc.) Allow a moment for reflection and then have the group begin sharing their names, beginning with a volunteer.

After the volunteer speaks, ask the next person in the circle to repeat the first name and then say her own. Continue moving around the circle in this fashion — each new speaker recites all the previous names in order and then adds his own to the end of the list.

It is probably best to explain the exercise completely before beginning so that the activity isn't interrupted by instructions. If the group consists of more than 20 people, it is helpful to split up into two smaller groups.

After the name-saying has passed all the way around the circle, invite a volunteer to attempt the entire list in reverse order for additional fun.

Just The Facts

In this exercise each participant chooses a personal detail to share and the group attempts to match facts with faces.

Give each person in the group a blank note card or similarly sized piece of paper and invite everyone to record, using a simple sentence, one factual but presumably unknown-to-the-group statement about their own lives. Collect all note cards, put them into one container, shuffle the contents well and then ask for a volunteer.

Have the volunteer draw one card (someone else's!), read it aloud and take a guess about who wrote the fact. If the guess is right, pass the fact container to the next person and repeat. If the first guess is incorrect, allow the entire group one guess as to the actual author and then ask the "owner" of the fact to reveal his or her identity before the next person takes a turn.

The Story of My Name
Initiating a dialogue about our cultural differences can be an important part of developing group trust. This activity, sharing the stories of our names, can foster the beginning of such discussions.

Arrange a writing surface — use large piece(s) of paper on an easel, a whiteboard, a chalkboard or a projector screen, for example — so that all participants can see it with ease. Have group members, one at a time, write, say aloud and then briefly tell the story of their full names.

Ask each person to share the answers to questions like: Where did your name come from? How was your name chosen for you? Does your name reflect the history of your family or culture of origin? Do you have a nickname that has grown from your given name?

Bibliography and Suggested Readings

Bibliography

de la Huerta, Christian. *Coming Out Spiritually: The Next Step.*
New York: Jeremy P. Tarcher/Putnam, 1999.

Flunder, Bishop Yvette A. *Where the Edge Gathers: Building a Community of Radical Inclusion.*
Cleveland, OH: The Pilgrim Press, 2005.

Hardy, Robin with David Groff. *The Crisis of Desire: AIDS and the Fate of Gay Brotherhood.*
Minneapolis: The University of Minnesota Press, 2002.

Lamott, Anne. *Traveling Mercies: Some Thoughts on Faith.*
New York, New York: Anchor Books, 1999.

Lamott, Anne. "Almost 86'd" *San Francisco Stories: Great Writers on the City,*
ed. John Miller. San Francisco: Chronicle Books LLC, 1990.

Lee, Dr. Steven J. *Overcoming Crystal Meth Addiction: An Essential Guide to Getting Clean.*
New York, New York: Marlowe & Company, 2006.

Merrill, Nan C. *Psalms for Praying.*
New York: Continuum International Publishing Group, 2007.

Messer, Donald E. *Breaking the Conspiracy of Silence: Christian Churches and the Global AIDS Crisis.*
Minneapolis, MN: Augsburg Fortress, Fortress Press, 2004.

Pieters, A. Stephen. *"I'm Still Dancing!" A Gay Man's Health Experience.*
Gaithersburg, MD: Chi Rho Press, 1991.

Pieters, Rev. Steve, Rev. Elder Don Eastman and Gary McClelland.
"CDC Broadens Definition of AIDS."
ALERT: News from MCC on Legislation, Education, Research and Treatment.
September 1987.

Priests for Equality, *The Inclusive Bible: The First Egalitarian Translation.*
United Kingdom: Sheed & Ward Book, 2007.

Rubin, Gayle. "Thinking Sex: Notes for a Radical Theory on the Politics of Sexuality."
Pleasure and Danger: Exploring Female Sexuality, ed. Carole S. Vance.
London: Pandora, 1992.

Sacks, Rabbi Johnathan. *To Heal a Fractured World: The Ethics of Responsibility.*
    New York: Schocken Books, 2005.

Selders, Jr., Bishop John. "Calling on Religious Leadership for World AIDS Day."
    World AIDS Day, 2007.

Shelp, Earl E. and Ronald H. Sunderland. *AIDS and the Church: The Second Decade.*
    Louisville, KY: Westminster / John Knox Press, 1992.

Sontag, Susan. *Illness as Metaphor and AIDS and Its Metaphors.*
    New York: Picador, 1990.

UNAIDS. *08 Report on the Global AIDS Epidemic: Executive Summary.*
    Geneva: UNAIDS, 2008.

Wilson, Rev. Elder Nancy. *Our Tribe: Queer Folks, God, Jesus, and the Bible.*
    Tajique, NM: Alamo Square Press, 1995.

World Council of Churches. *Facing AIDS: The Challenge, the Churches' Response.*
    Geneva: World Council of Churches, 1997.

Suggested Readings

Ariss, Robert M. *Against Death: The Practice of Living with AIDS.*
    Amsterdam: OPA (Overseas Publishers Association), 1997.

Behrman, Greg. *The Invisible People: How the U.S. Has Slept Through the Global*
    AIDS Pandemic, the Greatest Humanitarian Catastrophe of Our Time.
    New York: Free Press, Simon & Schuster, 2004.

Brand, Alan. *Positively Alive.*
    Johannesburg, South Africa: Jacana Media, 2005.

Brown, Rebecca. *The Gifts Of The Body.*
    New York: Harper Collins, 1994.

Burrow, Jr., Rufus. James H. *Cone and Black Liberation Theology.*
    Jefferson, North Carolina: McFarland, 2001.

D'Adesky, Anne-Christine. *Moving Mountains: The Race to Treat Global AIDS.*
    New York: Verso, 2004.

Eichberg, Rob. *Coming Out: An Act of Love.*
    New York: Plume, 1990.

Epperly, Bruce G. *Healing Worship: Purpose and Practice.*
    Cleveland, OH: The Pilgrim Press, 2006.

Fox, Matthew. *Wrestling with the Prophets: Essays on Creation Spirituality and Everyday Life.*
    San Francisco: HarperSanFrancisco, 1995.

Goss, Rev. Robert E. *Queering Christ: Beyond Jesus Acted Up.*
    Cleveland, OH: The Pilgrim Press, 2002.

Goss, Rev. Robert E. and Rev. Mona West, eds. *Take Back The Word: A Queer Reading of the Bible.*
    Cleveland, OH: The Pilgrim Press, 2000.

Holleran, Andrew. *Chronicle Of A Plague, Revisited: AIDS and its Aftermath.*
    New York: Da Capo Press, Perseus Books Group, 2008.

hooks, bell. *Feminism is for Everybody: Passionate Politics.*
    Cambridge, MA: South End Press, 2005.

hooks, bell. *Sisters of the Yam: black women and self-recovery.*
    Cambridge, MA: South End Press, 2005.

Itano, Nicole. *No Place Left To Bury The Dead: Denial, Despair, and Hope
    In the African AIDS Pandemic.*
    New York: Atria Books, Simon & Schuster, 2007.

Kavar, Louis F. *Families Re-Membered: Pastoral Support for Friends and Families Living
    with Hiv/Aids.*
    Gaithersburg, MD: Chi Rho Press, 1993.

Lake, Deborah. *Your Sister, Your Brother, Your Neighbor Has AIDS.*
    Chicago: Brush Arbor Press, 2006.

Loughlin, Gerard. *Queer Theology: Rethinking the Western Body.*
    Oxford, UK: Blackwell Publishing, 2007.

Lorde, Audre. *The Cancer Journals.*
    San Francisco, CA: Aunt Lute, 1997.

Nepo, Mark. *The Exquisite Risk: Daring to Live an Authentic Life.*
    New York: Three Rivers Press, 2005.

Patte, Daniel, General Ed. *Global Bible Commentary.*
    Nashville, Tennessee: Abingdon Press, 2004. "Mark's Healing Stories in an AIDS
    Context" Musa W. Dube.

Pearson, Bishop Carlton. *The Gospel of Inclusion: Reaching Beyond Religious Fundamentalism to the True Love of God.*
USA: AZUSA Press, 2006.

Perry, Rev. Elder Troy and Thomas L. P. Swicegood. *Don't Be Afraid Anymore.*
New York: St. Martin's Press, 1990.

Rieder, Ines and Patricia Ruppelt. *AIDS: The Women.*
Pittsburgh, PA: Cleis Press, 1988.

Robbins, Trina; Bill Sienkiewicz and Robert Triptow, eds.
Strip AIDS U.S.A.: A Collection of Cartoon Art To Benefit People With AIDS.
San Francisco: Last Gasp, 1988.

Rofes, Eric. *Reviving the Tribe: Regenerating Gay Men's Sexuality and Culture in the Ongoing Epidemic.*
Binghamton, NY: Harrington Park Press / The Haworth Press, Inc., 1995.

Rofes, Eric. *Dry Bones Breathe: Gay Men Creating Post-AIDS Identities and Cultures.*
Binghamton, NY: Harrington Park Press / The Haworth Press, Inc., 1998.

Sauers, Joan. *Sex Lives of Australian Teenagers.*
Sydney, Australia: Random House Australia, 2007.

Scare, Michael. *Smearing the Queer: Medical Bias in the Health Care of Gay Men.*
New York: Harrington Park Press / The Haworth Press, Inc., 1999.

Shilts, Randy. *And The Band Played On: Politics, People, And The AIDS Epidemic.*
New York: St. Martin's Press, 1988.

Smallman, Shawn. *The AIDS Pandemic in Latin America.*
Chapel Hill: The University Of North Carolina Press, 2007.

Spanbauer, Tom. *The City of Shy Hunters.*
New York: Grove Press, 2001.

Winick, Judd. *Pedro and Me: Friendship, Loss, and What I Learned.*
New York: Henry Holt and Company, 2000.

Acknowledgements

*This book has been a labor of love that grew from a multitude of relationships,
a lifetime of learning and teaching moments, and a huge amount of pure
faith that the limits of human communication are always translated and magnified
by the grace of God.*

*I endeavor here to reflect in some small way the "village" it has taken to raise this
ministry. Each of these people – and in truth so many unnamed – have taught me
about the* Uncommon Hope *that we have prayed into this ministry.*

*To my beloved family, of birth and choice, I offer the most precious gift I can
think to offer – my ongoing commitment to walk with God, to honor my call and to
love this world beyond measure – because of you.*
Uncle Patrick Herndon (in memorium); Mom (Cindi) and Sue; Hannah, Melanie; Bobby; Sissy; Trent,
Heather and Sailor; Rosana M.; Matt B.; Gina, Russell and Chris; Debra...and so many more.

To my mentors and teachers, I offer this:
*"Two roads diverged in a wood, and I – I took the one less traveled by,
And that has made all the difference."*   *Robert Frost*
Lynn Shepodd, National Coming Out Day; Matthew C. Brown, Ph.D., University of Colorado,
Boulder, Colorado; Rev. Lea Brown, MCC San Francisco; Rev. Pat Bumgardner, MCC New York;
Rev. Dr. Donald Messer, Center for the Church and Global AIDS; Eric Rofes (in memorium),
Gay Men's Health Movement; Chris Bartlett, Gay Men's Health Movement; Honey Ward, The Experience;
Rob Eichberg (in memorium), The Experience; Don P. (in memorium); Mark D. Jordan, Harvard
Divinity School; the amazing Faculty and Staff of Episcopal Divinity School; Matt Patrick,
Sarah Annecone and the staff and board of the Boulder County AIDS Project (1995-1996 and 2000-
2001); the incredible teaching congregation of MCC San Francisco...and all the many activists,
theologians, educators and workers who strive each day to make the world a better place.

*To the people who have been my friends in the face of my fierce determination
to make a change in the world. I pray that God gives me enough years to grow into
the person I hope to be and the friend you all deserve.*
Rosana Mina; Matt Brown; Jesse Stommel; Tina Tesch; Stephanie Smith; Jason O'Neil; Rev. Ellen
Richardson; Booth Towry-Iburg; Van English; Dr. Carol Kiesling; Connie Meadows;
Rev. Candy Holmes; Derek, Sue and Maya Cram-Mountain; Susan Canal; Scotty Embry; Scott Perkins;
Kathy Beasley and Valerie Parson; Ritchie Crownfield and Alan Landis; The Deegans; John Ekeberg;
Greg Geihsler; Jakob Hero; Brian Hutchison and James Schardin; Sarah Park; Justin Ritchie;
John McLaughlin; Rev. Gavin Ward; Dan Schellhorn(in memoriam); Rev. Delores Berry and
Judy Kiser; Dr. Paula (Auntie Paula) Schoenwether; Matt Bucy; and Bishop John Selders.

To the creative team who made this a real possibility – your ability to see around the corners of my mind and into the depths of my heart have made this a triumph for a community.

Leah Sloan, the world's best editor; Joe Rattan, for a design that captivates hearts and minds; Rev. Dr. Cindi Love, for resourcing this project from its conception; Melanie Martinez, for crafting an exceptional online presence and ministry; Jesse Stommel, the film editor and artist who helped me tell the story of children on the other side of the world with dignity and love; Christy Ebner, for hearing your own call to this ministry and caring for the lives we touched as if they were your own family; Rev. Elder Jim Mitulski, for your tenacious work to keep the "old songs" alive and for encouraging me to take my turn at leadership; Rev. Elder Ken Martin, for modeling for me the very picture of a servant leader and then letting me take flight; Rev. Elder Nancy Wilson, for passionately insisting that we remain a movement and ministry of justice, healing and love – no matter what; Rev. Elder Troy Perry, for committing every single moment of your life to transforming the world into a place where all of this work and so much more would be possible.

To my special angels

Rev. Marty Luna-Wolfe and Rev. Maria Luna-Wolfe

To the medical staff who have lovingly cared for me through these many years of living with HIV

Dr. Charles Steinberg; Dr. Ben Young; Dr. Michael Mohr; Rosa; Billy and Amy; Tara Kennedy, FNP; Dr. Rick Loftus

Moderators of Metropolitan Community Churches

Rev. Elder Troy Perry, Founder and 1st Moderator
Rev. Elder Nancy Wilson, Moderator
Rev. Elder Don Eastman, Vice Moderator, retired
Rev. Elder Darlene Garner, Vice Moderator and Region 6 Elder

Board of Elders of Metropolitan Community Churches

Rev. Elder Ken Martin, Region 1
Rev. Elder Arlene Ackerman, Region 3
Rev. Elder Glenna Shepherd, Region 4
Rev. Elder Diane Fisher, Region 5
Rev. Elder Lillie Brock, Region 7
Rev. Elder Jim Mitulski, (formerly) Region 2
Rev. Elder Debbi Martin, (formerly) Region 1
Rev. Elder Cecilia Eggleston, (formerly) Region 4

Board of Administration of Metropolitan Community Churches
Rev. Jeff Miner, Chair
Julie Krueger, Clerk
Marsha Warren, Treasurer
Marvin Bagwell
Barb Crabtree
John Vespa
John Hassell

Lay Ministry Council of Metropolitan Community Churches
Bryan Parker, Chair
Marsha Stevens-Pino, Vice-Chair
Charlene Bisordi
Paul Johnstone
Jan Miels
Randi Williams

Staff of Metropolitan Community Churches
Kathy Beasley, Rev. Dr. Sharon Bezner, Rev. Jim Birkitt, Florin Buhuceanu, Franklin Calvin, Carlos Chavez, Sharon Cox, Ritchie Crownfield, Angel Collie, Judy Dale, Christy Ebner, Rev. Karla Fleshman, Rev. Thomas Friedhoff, Vickey Gibbs, Rev. Jennifer Glass, Rev. Hector Gutierrez, Kay Hale, Bill Hooper, Jennifer Justice, Marina Laws, Irma Bauer-Levesque, Steve Marlowe, Melanie Martinez, Connie Meadows, Jason O'Neill, Valarie Parson, Stedney Phillips, Joseph (Joe) Rattan, Leah Sloan, Rev. Margaret Walker, Rev. Dr. Mona West, Frank Zerilli, ...and all the other members of the Team That Beats with One Heart.

The Fellowship
Bishop Yvette Flunder and Mother Shirley Miller
Roni Jordan
Rev. Kendal Brown
Rev. Jeffrey Campbell
Pastor Noni Gordon
Minister Franzetta Houston
Pastor Troy Sanders
...and so many others who have generously helped me to grow as a faith leader.

MCCGHAM Program Churches and Partner Organizations – 2005 to 2009

Exodus Metropolitan Community Church
Abilene, Texas, USA
Rev. Margaret Walker and Rev. Connie J. Mangin

Little River United Church of Christ
Annandale, Virginia, USA
Rev. James M. Bell

First Metropolitan Community Church of Atlanta
Atlanta, Georgia, USA
Rev. Paul Graetz and Steven Coughlin, Ph.D.

Open Door Metropolitan Community Church
Boyds, Maryland, USA
Rev. Rob Apgar-Taylor and Adam DeBaugh

General Conference and World Jubilee 2005
Calgary, Alberta, Canada
Rev. Paul Fairley (in memorium) and the Planning and Leadership Team

Metropolitan Community Church of Greater Dallas and AIDS Interfaith Network
Dallas, Texas, USA
Rev. Colleen Darraugh, Rev. Steven Pace, Rev. Cheryl Jordan

Metropolitan Community Church of the Rockies
Denver, Colorado, USA
Rev. Jim Burns, John Allison and Rick Smith

Center for Church and Global AIDS
Denver, Colorado, USA
Rev. Dr. Donald Messer

Metropolitan Community Church of Northern Virginia (NOVA)
Fairfax, Virginia, USA
Rev. Kharma Amos

Imago Dei Metropolitan Community Church
Glen Mills, Pennsylvania, USA
Rev. Karla Fleshman

Gay Men's Health Movement Leadership Academies of 2006 and 2008
Guerneville, California, USA
Eric Rofes, Chris Bartlett, T. Scott Pegues, Kevin Trimell Jones and Fred Lopez

Safe Harbour Metropolitan Community Church
Halifax, Nova Scotia, Canada
Rev. Darlene Young (in memorium), Bob Fougere and Sam Wilson

Metropolitan Community Church of the Spirit
Harrisburg, Pennsylvania, USA
Rev. Eva O'Diam

Spirit of Hope Metropolitan Community Church
Kansas City, Missouri, USA
Rev. John Barbone and Rev. Kurt Krieger

Lancaster Theological Seminary
Lancaster, Pennsylvania, USA
Rev. Dr. Bruce Epperly, Dr. David M. Mellott and Bryce Rich

New Covenant Metropolitan Community Church
Laurel, Maryland, USA
Rev. Lance F. Mullins

Metropolitan Community Church of Los Angeles
Los Angeles, California, USA
Rev. Neil G. Thomas, Rev. Pat Langlois and Rev. Alejandro Escoto

Metropolitan Community Church Melbourne
Melbourne, Victoria, Australia
Rev. Heather Creighton and Jan Miels

AIDS 2008 - International AIDS Conference
Mexico City, Mexico

AIDS 2008 - Ecumenical Pre-Conference, "Faith in Action Now!"
Mexico City, Mexico
The Ecumenical Advocacy Alliance (EAA)

All God's Children Metropolitan Community Church
Minneapolis, Minnesota, USA
Rev. Paul Ecknes-Tucker, Rev. Robyn Provis

Pride Institute - LGBT Mental Health and Chemical Dependency Care
Minneapolis, Minnesota, USA
Pablo McCabe, Donna Gimbut and Marty Perry

Vision of Hope Metropolitan Community Church and Ribbons of Hope Support Group
Mountville, Pennsylvania, USA
Rev. Debbie Coggin and Rev. Jennifer Glass; Chris Jackson, Tom Buzak, Bev Bauer, Russ Baker, Fean Rogers, Jeff Roane and Mykal Slack

Metropolitan Community Church of New York
New York, New York, USA
Rev. Pat Bumgardner, Rev. Edgard Danielsen-Morales, Rev. Boon Ngeo, Bradley Curry, Noah Seaton, Lucky S. Michaels, William Moran-Berberena

Metropolitan Community Church of Omaha
Omaha, Nebraska, USA
Rev. Tom Emmett and Troy Fienhold-Haasis

MCC of the Palm Beaches
Palm Beach Gardens, Florida, USA
Rev. Paul Whiting and Karl Zwarych

MCC Portland
Portland, Oregon, USA
Rev. Glenna Shepherd, Rev. Wes Mullins, Rev. Dianne Shaw, Mark Brown, Steven Couch, Chris Culver

LGBTI Health Summit of Philadelphia
Philadelphia, Pennsylvania, USA
Bill Jesdale, Chris Bartlett and the planning teams

MCC Regions 3 and 5 - Regional Conference
Pittsburgh, Pennsylvania, USA
Conference Planning Teams

City of Refuge United Church of Christ
San Francisco, California, USA
Bishop Yvette Flunder and Mother Shirley Miller; and the many faithful ministers and lovers
of God at C.O.R and Refuge Ministries

MCC San Francisco
San Francisco, California, USA
Rev. Dr. G. Penny Nixon, Rev. Charles Tigard, Stephanie Smith, Rev. Jill Sizemore,
MCCSF Board and Staff

Church of the Trinity MCC
Sarasota, Florida, USA
Rev. Dr. Mona West, Rev. David S. Wynn, Paul DiPlacido, Hope Wulliman and all the many
servant leaders in the pews of this church.

Regions 1, 6 and 7 Regional Conference
Scottsdale, Arizona, USA
Conference Planning Team

General Conference and World Jubilee 2007
Scottsdale, Arizona, USA
Conference Planning Team: Christy Ebner, Rev. Alejandro Escoto, Rev. Karen Ziegler,
Rev. Elder Jim Mitulski, Rev. Elder Freda Smith, Rev. Elder Hong Tan, Rev. Nokthula Dhladhla,
Rev. Paul Mokgethi, Rev. Hector Gutierrez, Nessette Falu, Eve Plews, Mark Kruse

MCC of Greater St. Louis and The Ezekiel Project
St. Louis, Missouri, USA
Rev. Dr. Carol Trissell, Rev. Sue Yarber, Rev. Dale Chavis, Danny Gladden, Rev. Jeff Bert,
Keith Richardson and Chuck VanHorn

MCC Good Shepherd
Granville, New South Wales, Australia
Rev. Robert Clark, Rev. Gavin Ward and Robert Ryan

MCC Sydney
Sydney, New South Wales, Australia
Rev. Karl Hand

MCC of Tampa
Tampa, Florida, USA
Rev. Phyllis Hunt, Rev. David Gant, Vilia Corvison and Mac McGowan

MCC Toronto
Toronto, Ontario, Canada
Rev. Dr. Brent Hawkes; Rev. Jo Bell; Deacon Sandra Millar, Robert Dykeman and the amazing staff and congregation there.

Metropolitan Community Church of Washington, DC
Washington, D.C., USA
Rev. Dr. Candace Shultis, Rev. Mark Byrd, Rev. Reg Richburg

Wichita Falls MCC and No Day But Today
Wichita Falls, Texas, USA
Rev. Lea Brown, John Forsythe, Neal Goerz

MCC of Winston-Salem
Winston-Salem, North Carolina, USA
Rev. Joe Cobb and Randy Burchette

Press

The East County Observer
Sarasota, Florida, USA
Kristie A. Martinez

Halifax Daily News
Halifax, Nova Scotia, Canada
Jon Tattrie, writer

International Association of Physicians in AIDS Care (IAPAC+)
Global

National Public Radio
Mexico City, Mexico
Michael O'Boyle

Sex Smarts, Campus Radio 1190, University of Colorado, Boulder, Colorado
Hosted by Matthew C. Brown, Ph.D.

Wayves
Halifax, Nova Scotia, Canada
Bill McKinnon, writer

Well, Well, Well on JOY 94.9
Melbourne, Victoria, Australia
Tex McKenzie

MCCGHAM Sponsors and Major Donors
Elton John AIDS Foundation
Rainbow Endowment
Martina Navratilova
Barbara Delaney, CEO of Navratilova Inc.
Ann Vassilaros and Fran Solitro
Mitchell Gold, Co-Founder and Chairman, The Mitchell Gold Co.
Steve Coughlin, Ph.D.
Tseli Mohammed, The Leadership Campaign on AIDS
John "Jack" Miller
Rev. Dr. Cindi Love and Sue Jennings
Miguel Gomez, Director, AIDS.gov, US Department of Health and Human Services (HHS)
Dan Schellhorn
Sherrill Parmley

Special Colleagues in the Struggle to Make Change a Reality
John D. Hassell, UNAIDS; Pauline Muchina, UNAIDS; Jewish Mosaic - Gregg Drinkwater and
David Shneer; Amber Hollibaugh, formerly of the National Gay and Lesbian Taskforce; Harry Knox,
Human Rights Campaign; Rev. Rebecca Voelkel, National Gay and Lesbian Taskforce; Ann Craig,
GLAAD; Rev. Michael Schuenemeyer, United Church of Christ Global HIV/AIDS Ministry;
Rev. Ruth Garwood, The UCC Coalition for LGBT Concerns; Christian de la Huerta; Tex McKenzie;
Rev. Elisabeth Middelberg and Cindy Acker; Rev. Terri Echelbarger; Rev. Dan Koeshall;
Rev. Nathan Meckley; Rev. Wes Mullins; Rev. Jim Merritt, Al Leach, John Munera; Rev. Joe McMurray;
Rev. Elder Nori Rost; Rev. David Mundy; Rev. Michelle Kirby; Rev. Durrell Watkins;
Rev. Roland Stringfellow; Lynn Jordan, MCCSF Archives Project; Miguel Gomez, HHS/OPHS;
International Association of Physicians in AIDS Care (IAPAC+)

MCCGHAM, Past Leadership
Rev. Steve Pieters
Rev. David Farrell
Rev. Robert Griffin
Rev. Elder Hong Tan
Rev. Elder Jim Mitulski
Christy Ebner

Any omissions and misspellings are inadvertent and regretted.

Photo Identification and Credits

Cover

Upper left: A child praying at Mother of Peace Orphanage in Zimbabwe; photo by members of the delegation who visited Mother of Peace in 2006

Upper right: Kathy Beasley; photo courtesy of Kathy Beasley

Lower right: Christy Ebner and a child of Mother of Peace Orphanage; photo by members of the delegation who visited Mother of Peace in 2007

Lower left: Joshua L. Love at MCC General Conference 2005; photo by Stephanie Houfek

Center: Marchers in the Inaugural International March Against Homophobia, Stigmatization & Discrimination in Mexico City, 2008; photo by Rev. Dr. Donald Messer

Table of Contents

Marchers; photo by Rev. Dr. Donald Messer

Foreword

Photo supplied by Rev. Dr. Donald Messer

Author's Note

Photo by Paula Fraser

Introduction

(from l. to r.)

Rev. Paul Mokgethi, Hope & Unity MCC of Johannesburg, South Africa, at the International AIDS Conference, 2008; photo by Bobby G. Pierce

A marcher at the Inaugural International March Against Homophobia, Stigmatization & Discrimination; photo by Bobby G. Pierce

Joshua L. Love and a baby of Mother of Peace Orphanage; photo by Christy Ebner

Melinda Cochran, MCCGHAM supporter; photo by Kristine Poggioli, *www.NonProfitCopy.com*

Chronology

p. 13, l to r: C. Bruce Bunger; photo from the MCC San Francisco archives

Joshua L. Love and Baby Anthony; photo by members of the delegation who visited Mother of Peace in 2006

Children's graves at Mother of Peace Orphanage; photo by members of the delegation who visited Mother of Peace in 2006

p. 14: Rev. Steve Pieters; MCC Archives photo from his appearance on Tammy Faye Bakker's television show

p.15: Rev. David Farrell; photo from the MCC archives

p.16: A hand-beaded AIDS ribbon from South Africa; photo by Joshua L. Love

p.17: Memorial panels of Frank Koelling and David Zink, congregants at MCC of Greater St. Louis in St. Louis, Missouri, USA; photos by Ritchie Crownfield

p.19: Jack's handprint, Melbourne, Victoria, Australia, 2007; photo by Joshua L. Love

p.20: Sister Unity of the Sisters of Perpetual Indulgence at MCC Los Angeles, World AIDS Day 2002; photo by Mark S. Hahn

p.23: James Boyd and James Lin, MCCGHAM supporters; photo by Kristine Poggioli

p. 25 Chris Freimuth and Rev. Lea Brown, MCCGHAM supporters; photo by Kristine Poggioli

p.26: Ritchie Crownfield, Rev. Elder Jim Mitulski and Joshua L. Love at MCC of Greater St. Louis, AIDS Retreat Weekend, May 2006; photo by Rev. Dale Chavis

p. 27 Melanie Martinez, MCC staff and MCCGHAM supporter, photo by Lynn Michelle Photography, 2007

p. 29 Yew Hoe Tan, MCCGHAM supporter; photo by Kristine Poggioli

p.30: Rev. Elder Ken Martin and Joshua L. Love, Melbourne, 2007; photo by Rev. Heather Creighton

Chapter 1

p.32: World image by Cartesia from PhotoDisc/Global Perspectives disc no. 17

p.38: Rev. Kharma Amos and Joshua L. Love; photo by Christy Ebner

Chapter 2

p.76: Torso; photo courtesy of Jesse Stommel

p.81, l to r: Sue Parcel, MCCGHAM supporter; photo by Kristine Poggioli

      Lewis & Maxwell Reay, MCCGHAM supporters; photo by Stephanie Houfek

      Jubilee Jee and Pam Quiton, MCCGHAM supporters; photo by Kristine Poggioli

      Aiden Dunn, MCCGHAM supporter; photo courtesy of A. Dunn

p.82, l to r: Child at Mother of Peace; photo by members of the delegation who visited Mother of Peace in 2007

      Bobby G. Pierce, MCCGHAM supporter; photo by Rev. Dr. Donald Messer

      Cheri Toney, MCCGHAM supporter; photo by Christine Poggioli

      Rev. Lance Mullins, MCCGHAM supporter; photo by Christy Ebner

Chapter 3

p.86: "Don't Forget Us"; taken at Sylvia's Place

p.91: above, youth at Sylvia's Place

      below, the cover of Lucky S. Michaels's book *Shelter*. Trolley Books, 2008.

p.93: "Charlene" from Shelter. This image appeared in the *New York Times*.

p.94: Benji in "No Girls Allowed" from *Shelter*

      All the photographs in this chapter are by and used with the permission of Lucky S. Michaels

Chapter 4

p.120: A poster at Mother of Peace; photo by members of the delegation who visited Mother of Peace in 2007

p.122, t to b: Paul Hufstedler, MCCGHAM supporter; photo by Kristine Poggioli

      Rahn Anderson, Greg Carey and Will Dounley, MCCGHAM supporters; photo by Kristine Poggioli

      Jack Hubbs, Diane Kalliam and Ms. Eva Lily, MCCGHAM supporters; photo by Kristine Poggioli

      Ilyas Ilya, MCCGHAM supporter; photo by Kristine Poggioli

p.124, l to r: Angel Collie, MCC staff member and MCCGHAM supporter; photo by Stephanie Houfek

      Carolyn Eidson and Kristine Poggioli, MCCGHAM supporters; photo courtesy of K. Poggioli

p.125, l to r: Troy Brunet, MCCGHAM supporter; photo by Kristine Poggioli

      Francisco Caravayo, MCCGHAM supporter MCCGHAM supporter; photo by Kristine Poggioli

p.127: Images from the May 2006 AIDS Retreat Weekend at MCC of Greater St. Louis; photos by Ritchie Crownfield

p.128: Images from the May 2006 AIDS Retreat Weekend at MCC of Greater St. Louis; photos by Ritchie Crownfield

Chapter 5

p.132: Joshua L. Love beside one of the "Y Sculptures" in Cambridge Parks; photo by Bobby G Pierce

p.134: A poster advertising a candlelight march; photo courtesy of MCC San Francisco

p.136, l to r: Joshua L. Love on World AIDS Day, 2008; photo by Bobby G. Pierce

      The altar at MCC San Francisco on World AIDS Day, 2008; photo by Bobby G. Pierce

p137, l to r: At MCC San Francisco on World AIDS Day, 2008; photo by Bobby G. Pierce

      A display of Ribbons of Hope at Visions of Hope MCC in Mountville, Pennsylvania (USA) on World AIDS Day, 2007; photo by Christy Ebner

Chapter 6

All of the photographs in this chapter were lovingly taken by members of the delegations who visited Mother of Peace Orphanage in Zimbabwe in 2006 and 2007.

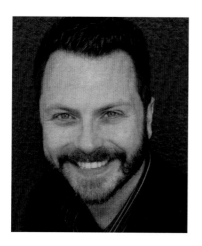

Joshua L. Love

Joshua L. Love, director of the Metropolitan
Community Churches Global HIV/AIDS Ministry
(MCCGHAM) and Metropolitan Community
Churches Drug and Addictions Ministry is a passionate
advocate for LGBTIQ health and wellness. Joshua,
a survivor of HIV and drug addiction, travels the world
to share a message of hope and spiritual renewal
as well as his personal experiences as he works to further
the development of community dialogues. He is a
clergy candidate, has been published in *IAPAC+*, and has
produced a documentary. Joshua's combination of
personal narrative and community dialogue brings light
to a set of challenging social and spiritual topics.

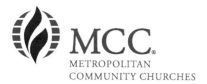

METROPOLITAN
COMMUNITY CHURCHES

**Tearing Down Walls
Building Up Hope**

**1500 Industrial Boulevard
Abilene, Texas USA 79602**

**P.O. Box 1374
Abilene, Texas USA 79604**

1.866.HOPE.MCC

www.mccchurch.org